OPERATIVE ANATOMY
of THORAX

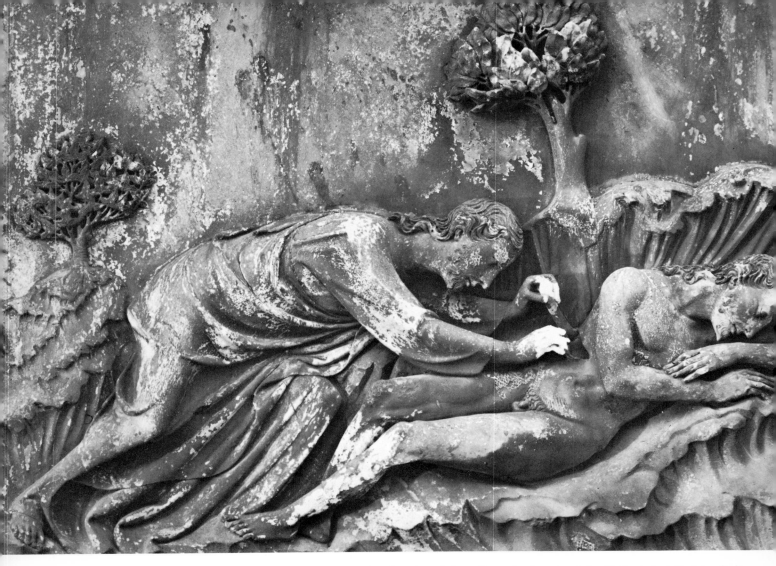

The Creation of Eve. *From the façade of the Cathedral of Orvieto, Italy. Attributed to Giovanni Pisano.* (Courtesy of Dr. Edward D. Churchill.)

Edward A. Edwards, M.D.

Surgeon, Peter Bent Brigham Hospital. Clinical Professor of Anatomy, Harvard Medical School.

Paul D. Malone, A.B.

Director of Medical Illustration, Lahey Clinic Foundation. Member, Association of Medical Illustrators.

John J. Collins, Jr., M.D.

Chief, Division of Thoracic and Cardiac Surgery, Peter Bent Brigham Hospital. Assistant Professor of Surgery, Harvard Medical School.

OPERATIVE ANATOMY of THORAX

LEA & FEBIGER Philadelphia

1972

ISBN 0-8121-0371-8
Published in Great Britain by Henry Kimpton Publishers, London

Library of Congress Catalog Card Number: 79-175458

Printed in the United States of America

preface

In calling this present work an 'operative anatomy,' the authors mean to focus on specific operative approaches, views seen at operation, anatomic anomalies to be expected, and operative dangers. Further, clinical evidence is adduced that may influence the surgeon in choosing alternatives in approaches and procedures. These aims would seem to make this book one on surgical technique, but the emphasis here is on what structures to find, how to find them, and what to avoid rather than on maneuver. It is planned to cover the entire body in this and subsequent volumes. The thorax was chosen for the first volume because it is felt that for this region, more than for others, available anatomy texts have failed to keep pace with the rapidly expanding needs of the surgeon.

The work rests heavily on a series of illustrations, but possesses more text than usually embellishes an atlas. No attempt is made to describe all structures comprehensively. We leave this task to a general textbook of anatomy. The presentation is regional, but modified by discussion and views of specific operations. The illustrations are partly original and partly taken from the literature, representing outstanding presentations of surgeons active in specific fields. We are greatly indebted to these individuals for the excellence of their publications and their generosity in allowing reproduction of their material.

Although we have attempted a comprehensive consideration of the anatomy of thoracic surgery, we have accepted a certain unevenness of emphasis. Thus we have presented the anatomy of the commonest of procedures for congenital heart disease, which could be understood without extensive study of the pathology of this category of disease. In general, views of operations of considerable scope have been chosen, the better to illustrate the anatomy of a part.

We thank our colleagues, young and old, for stimulation and advice. We are grateful to Professor Francis D. Moore for providing funds from the Surgical Department of the Peter Bent Brigham Hospital to help defray the expenses of this enterprise, and to Professor Don W. Fawcett for making available the facilities of the Department of Anatomy of the Harvard Medical School.

EDWARD A. EDWARDS
PAUL D. MALONE

Boston, Massachusetts   JOHN J. COLLINS, JR.

CONTENTS

SECTION 1
SUPERIOR APERTURE AND THORACIC WALL

Chapter 1. Superior Aperture   3

    Major Relationships at the Superior Aperture   3
    Removal of the First Rib for Relief of Neurovascular
        Compression   6

Chapter 2. Thoracic Wall   10

    Posterolateral Thoracoplasty   10
    Extrafascial Apicolysis   13
    Removal of Internal Thoracic Lymph Nodes   15
    Sympathectomy   16
        Cervicothoracic Sympathectomy   16
        Thoracolumbar Sympathectomy   20

SECTION 2
THE MEDIASTINUM EXCLUSIVE OF THE HEART AND PERICARDIUM

Chapter 3. The Mediastinum   29

    Boundaries and Contents   29
    Mediastinotomy and Mediastinoscopy   33

Chapter 4. Normal Variations in Branches of the Aortic Arch   40

    Patterns of Origin of the Major Arteries   40
    Variations of Origin of the Vertebral Arteries   41

Chapter 5. Exposures of the Aorta and Great Vessels   44

    Thoracic Exposures   44
    Exposure Extended to the Neck   47
    Cervico-axillary Extensions of Sternotomy   49

Chapter 6. Congenital Abnormalities of the Great Vessels   53

    Derivation of Anomalies of the Aorta and of Vascular
        Rings   53
    Vascular Rings   56
    Patent Ductus Arteriosus   57
    Coarctation of the Aorta   58

Chapter 7. Vascular Supply of the Thoracic Viscera, Exclusive
of the Coronary and Pulmonary Vessels   63

    Main Arterial Sources   63
    The Intercostal Arteries   64
    The Bronchial Arteries   65
    Arteries to Esophagus and Trachea   70
    Visceral Veins   72
    The Vascular Supply of the Spinal Cord   73

Chapter 8. Thoracic Aspects of Thyroid, Parathyroids, and Thymus   78

    Intrathoracic Goiter   78
    The Thyroidea Ima Artery   80
    The Retro-esophageal Subclavian Artery and the
        Inferior Laryngeal Nerve   81
    Intrathoracic Parathyroid Tumors   83
    Thymus   85

SECTION 3

The Heart and Pericardium

Chapter 9. Median Sternotomy   93

    Exposure   93
    Views of Pericardium, Thymus, Heart, and Major
        Vessels   95

Chapter 10. Right-sided Approach to the Atria; Mitral-Valve
Replacement   **100**

        Pericardial Attachment to the Great Veins   100
        Mitral-Valve Replacement   102
        The Cardiac Skeleton and Atrioventricular Perimeter   103

Chapter 11. Exposure of Mitral Valve from the Left; The Aortic
Valve   **108**

        Interior of Left Atrium and Ventricle   108
        Exposure of the Aortic Valve   110
        Anomalous Left Superior Vena Cava and Retro-
            aortic Left Brachiocephalic Vein   111

Chapter 12. Right Atrium and Ventricle   **115**

        Interior of the Right Atrium and Ventricle   115
        The Ventricular Musculature   118
        Valvular Variations and Networks in the Right Atrium   119

Chapter 13. Congenital Heart Disease   **124**

        Three Common Cardiac Defects   124
        Minor Variations of the Coronary Arteries   126
        Major Variations of the Coronary Arteries   127

Chapter 14. The Cardiac Conduction System   **132**

        Location of Major Components   132
        Intentional Interruption of Conduction Pathways   136

Chapter 15. Cardiac Transplantation   **138**

Chapter 16. The Coronary Arteries and Veins; Cardiac
Revascularization   **141**

        Patterns of Coronary Artery Distribution   141
        Blood Supply to the Atria and Nodal Tissue   144
        Natural External Collaterals for the Coronary System   146
        The Coronary Venous Sinus   147
        Myocardial Revascularization   149

Chapter 17. Cardiac Innervation   **153**

Chapter 18. Lymphatics of the Heart   **159**

Chapter 19. Pericardiocentesis and Drainage   162

     Approaches   162

     Pericardiectomy for Effusion   164

SECTION 4

LUNGS AND TRACHEA

Chapter 20. Pulmonary Lobes and Segments; Bronchoscopy   167

     Lobes and Fissures   167

     Segments   169

     Bronchoscopy   170

Chapter 21. The Lung Pedicle and Pulmonary Resections   173

     The Root of the Lung   173

     Major Lymphatic Trunks and Nodes   180

     Radical Pneumonectomy   183

     Intrahilar Anatomy and Lobar or Segmental Resection   184

Chapter 22. The Trachea   192

     Exposure   192

     Resection   193

SECTION 5

Thoracoabdominal Structures

Chapter 23. Visceral Topography and Exposures   199

     Subphrenic Visceral Relationships   199

     Thoracoabdominal Incisions   205

     Avoidance of Phrenic Nerve Injury   206

Chapter 24. Diaphragmatic and Hiatus Hernia   208

     Congenital Diaphragmatic Hernia   208

     Hiatus Hernia   210

       Operations for Hiatus Hernia   215

Chapter 25. Resection and Replacement of the Esophagus   218

    General Considerations   218

    Structures Employed for Bypass Grafting or
      Replacement   219

    Low Thoracic Esophagectomy and Esophagogastric
      Anastomosis   222

    High Thoracic Esophagectomy and Right-Sided
      Approaches   225

    Extrapleural Approaches to the Thoracic Esophagus   226

Chapter 26. The Thoracic Duct   228

    Usual Pattern of the Thoracic Duct and Its
      Tributaries   228

    Variations   229

    Collaterals for the Thoracic Duct   231

    Exposures of the Thoracic Duct and Cisterna Chyli   231

Index   235

illustrations

SECTION 1

Superior Aperture and Thoracic Wall

Figure 1.	Neurovascular relationships at the first rib.	4
Figure 2.	Structures at the apex of the pleura.	5
Figure 3.	The suprapleural membrane.	5
Figure 4.	Removal of the first rib through the axilla.	7
Figure 5.	Fasciae enclosing the pectoral and subclavius muscles.	8
Figure 6.	Posterolateral thoracoplasty.	11
Figure 7.	Deep upper parascapular structures.	12
Figure 8.	Costovertebral junctions and related anterior structures.	13
Figure 9.	Extrafascial apicolysis.	14
Figure 10.	Internal thoracic vessels and lymph nodes.	14
Figure 11.	Removal of sternocostal flap in extended radical mastectomy.	15
Figure 12.	Stellate ganglion and origin of the brachial plexus.	17
Figure 13.	Supraclavicular approach for cervicothoracic sympathectomy.	18–19
Figure 14.	Transthoracic and subdiaphragmatic extrapleural sympathectomy and splanchnicectomy.	20–21
Figure 15.	Transthoracic and transdiaphragmatic sympathectomy and splanchnicectomy.	22–23

SECTION 2

The Mediastinum Exclusive of the Heart and Pericardium

| Figure 16. | Right view of mediastinum and root of the lung. | 30 |
| Figure 17. | Left view of mediastinum and root of the lung. | 31 |

Figure 18. Cross sections of the mediastinum.   32
Figure 19. Extrapleural drainage of the superior
            mediastinum by cervical mediastinotomy.   34
Figure 20. Extrapleural drainage of the posterior
            mediastinum.   35
Figure 21. Cervicomediastinal exploration.   36–37
Figure 22. Mediastinal biopsy via the right second
            costal cartilage.   37
Figure 23. Variations in branching of the aortic arch.   41
Figure 24. Variations in origin and course of the
            vertebral arteries.   43
Figure 25. Exposure for subclavian–pulmonary artery
            anastomosis.   46
Figure 26. Extrapleural exposure of origin of left
            subclavian artery and sympathetic trunk.   47
Figure 27. Cervicothoracic exposure by bilateral
            sternoclavicular elevation.   49
Figure 28. Cervicothoracic exposure by
            sternoclavicular-pectoral pedicle.   50
Figure 29. Cervicothoracic-axillary exposure.   51
Figure 30. Aortic arches of mammalian embryo.   54
Figure 31. Derivation of aorta and vascular rings.   55
Figure 32. Division of vascular ring.   56
Figure 33. Exposure of patent ductus arteriosus.   58
Figure 34. Collateral circulation in coarctation of
            the aorta.   59
Figure 35. Posterolateral exposure for coarctation of
            the aorta.   60
Figure 36. Anterolateral exposure for coarctation of
            the aorta.   61
Figure 37. Sites of origin of 'Abbott's artery.'   61
Figure 38. Plan of the intercostal arteries.   65
Figure 39. Visceral branches of an intercostal artery.   66
Figure 40. Bronchial and esophageal arteries,
            right view.   67
Figure 41. Bronchial and esophageal arteries,
            left view.   68
Figure 42. Anomalous right bronchial artery.   69
Figure 43. Bronchial arteries and bronchial–pulmonary
            artery communications.   70
Figure 44. Venous drainage of the esophagus.   73
Figure 45. Vessels of the human spinal cord.   75
Figure 46. Cervicothoracic exposure for cancer of the
            thyroid.   79
Figure 47. Thyroidea ima artery arising from the
            brachiocephalic trunk.   80
Figure 48. Thyroidea ima artery arising from the arch
            of the aorta.   81
Figure 49. Descending course of inferior laryngeal
            nerve with retro-esophageal right sub-
            clavian artery.   82

Figure 50. Retro-esophageal right subclavian artery with anomalous origin of common carotid and the right vertebral artery. 83

Figure 51. Recurrence of the left inferior laryngeal nerve with right aortic arch and retro-esophageal left subclavian artery. 84

Figure 52. Paths of developmental migration, or adult displacement, of parathyroid adenomas. 84

Figure 53. The thymus in a newborn. 85

Figure 54. Thymic rests. 86

Figure 55. Vascular supply of the thymus. 87

SECTION 3

The Heart and Pericardium

Figure 56. Median sternotomy. 94

Figure 57. Lines of pleural reflection. 96

Figure 58. The posterior pericardium. 98

Figure 59. Right-sided exposure of the atria and the mitral valve. 101

Figure 60. The skeleton of the heart. 103

Figure 61. Structures in the atrioventricular perimeter. 104

Figure 62. Interior of the left ventricle. 105

Figure 63. Circumferences of the heart valves. 106

Figure 64. Interior of the left atrium and ventricle; exposure of aortic and mitral valves. 109

Figure 65. Anomalous left superior vena cava. 112

Figure 66. Two examples of retro-aortic left brachiocephalic vein. 113

Figure 67. Interior of the right atrium and ventricle. 116

Figure 68. The ventricular musculature. 119

Figure 69. Embryology of the venous valves of the right atrium. 120

Figure 70. Valvular variations and networks in the right atrium. 121

Figure 71. Three common congenital cardiac defects. 125

Figure 72. Intramural course of coronary arteries. 126

Figure 73. Anomalies of the coronary arteries. 128

Figure 74. Abnormal coronary artery communications. 129

Figure 75. The conduction system of the heart. 133

Figure 76. Transplantation of the heart. 139

Figure 77. Reciprocal relationship between the coronary arteries. 142

Figure 78. Anterior view of coronary distribution of 'balanced' type. 142

Figure 79. Posterior view of coronary distribution of 'balanced' type. 143

Figure 80. Posterior view of a 'left preponderant' coronary distribution. 143

Figure 81.   Arteries to the sinu-atrial node.   144
Figure 82.   The sinu-atrial node artery as a branch of
             a bronchial artery.   145
Figure 83.   The coronary venous system.   148
Figure 84.   Myocardial revascularization by intramural
             placement of the internal thoracic vessels.   150
Figure 85.   Cardiac branches from the cervical and
             thoracic sympathetic trunk.   154
Figure 86.   The cardiac plexus.   155
Figure 87.   Lymphatics of the heart.   160
Figure 88.   Pericardial puncture, drainage, and excision. 163

SECTiON 4

LuNqs ANd TRAChEA

Figure 89.   Pulmonary lobes and segments.   168
Figure 90.   Azygos lobe.   169
Figure 91.   Lobar and segmental bronchi.   171
Figure 92.   Right view of mediastinum and root of
             the lung.   174
Figure 93.   Left view of mediastinum and root of
             the lung.   175
Figure 94.   Typical branching of chief bronchi and
             blood vessels, right lung.   176
Figure 95.   Typical branching of chief bronchi and
             blood vessels, left lung.   177
Figure 96.   Artery to sequestered lung.   178
Figure 97.   Intrapericardial course of pulmonary veins.   179
Figure 98.   Pulmonary lymphatics: overall view.   180
Figure 99.   Pulmonary lymphatics: regional nodes.   181
Figure 100. Right radical pneumonectomy: early stage
             of dissection.   182
Figure 101. Right radical pneumonectomy: late stage
             of dissection.   183
Figure 102. Start of left radical pneumonectomy.   184
Figure 103. Hilum of right lung: anterior view.   185
Figure 104. Hilum of right lung: fissure view.   186
Figure 105. Hilum of right lung: posterior view.   187
Figure 106. Hilum of left lung: anterior view.   188
Figure 107. Hilum of left lung: fissure view.   189
Figure 108. Hilum of left lung: posterior view.   189
Figure 109. Lingulectomy.   190
Figure 110. Cervical tracheo-esophageal arteries.   193
Figure 111. Plans for resection of trachea.   194

SECTION 5
Thoracoabdominal Structures

Figure 112. Relations of viscera to the skeleton:
anterior view. 200
Figure 113. Relations of viscera to the skeleton:
posterior view. 201
Figure 114. Relations of viscera to the skeleton:
right lateral view. 202
Figure 115. Relations of viscera to the skeleton:
left lateral view. 203
Figure 116. Subphrenic peritoneal relationships. 204
Figure 117. Approaches to the subphrenic and
subhepatic spaces. 205
Figure 118. Phrenic nerve branching and diaphragmatic
incisions. 206
Figure 119. The diaphragm. 209
Figure 120. Types of diaphragmatic hernia. 210
Figure 121. Physiologic divisions of the distal
esophagus. 211
Figure 122. Role of muscle sling in sphincteric
function. 212
Figure 123. Varieties of hiatus hernia. 213
Figure 124. Thoracic repair of esophageal hiatus hernia. 214
Figure 125. Abdominal repair of hiatus hernia. 215
Figure 126. Esophageal bypass by subcutaneous
pedicled jejunogastrostomy. 220
Figure 127. Esophageal bypass by retrosternal pedicled
esophago-ileocolic-gastrostomy. 221
Figure 128. Replacement of cervical esophagus by free
graft of sigmoid colon with vascular
anastomosis. 222
Figure 129. Thoracic esophagectomy. 223
Figure 130. Esophagogastrostomy. 224
Figure 131. Extrapleural approach to esophageal atresia
and tracheo-esophageal fistula. 225
Figure 132. Variations of the thoracic duct. 229
Figure 133. Termination of the thoracic duct. 230
Figure 134. Transthoracic ligation of the cisterna chyli. 232

SECTION 1

Superior Aperture and Thoracic Wall

SUPERIOR APERTURE

MAJOR RELATIONSHIPS AT THE SUPERIOR APERTURE

The superior aperture of the thorax gives passage on each side to the apex of the lung and pleura and the neurovascular pedicle of the upper limb; medially it gives passage to the vessels of the head and neck and the midline viscera. Extrapleural relationships in this region are of special interest.

The first rib is a major surgical guide, its semicircle bounding the apex. The scalenus anterior muscle, inserting at about its middle, separates the subclavian vein in front from the subclavian artery and the trunks of the brachial plexus behind (Fig. 1). Posterior to the artery and nerves lies the scalenus medius muscle, also inserting on the first rib.

The first rib is atypical in having a flat cross section, with a sharp medial edge. The edge can easily be palpated at the neck of the rib, where the two nerve 'roots' (anterior rami of the eighth cervical and the first thoracic nerve) converge to form the inferior trunk of the brachial plexus, which lies on the rib behind the artery. In half of all subjects a scalenus minimus muscle, usually slender, is present, separating the artery from the inferior trunk of the plexus. The large stellate ganglion lies on the head of the first rib, with the costocervical trunk closer to the neck of the rib, and the vertebral artery and vein located more medially (Figs. 1 and 2).

The entire medial edge of the rib gives attachment to the suprapleural membrane (Sibson's fascia) (Fig. 3). The membrane is part of the endothoracic fascia, which bears

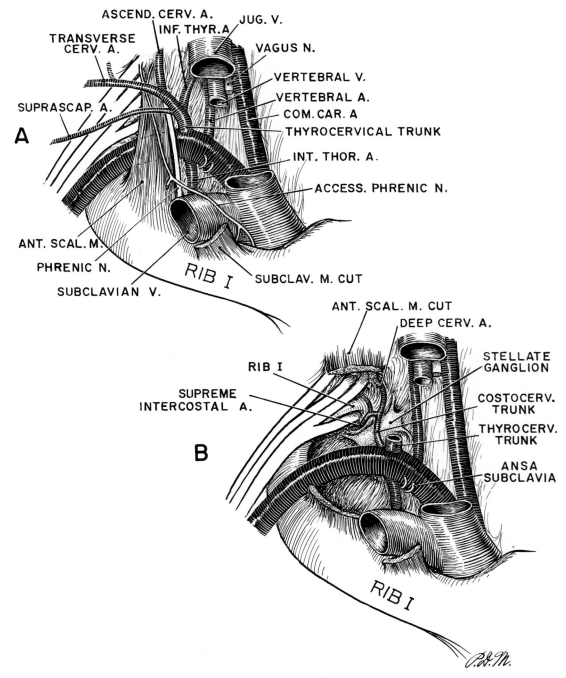

FIG. 1
Neurovascular relationships at the first rib. A. With scalenus anterior muscle intact; B, with muscle divided.

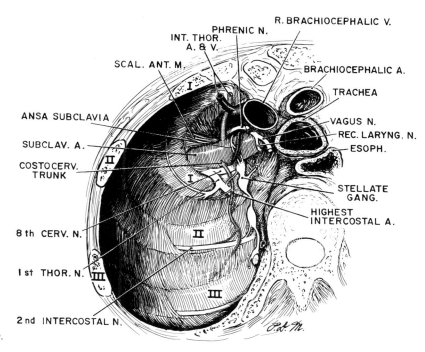

FIG. 2
Structures at the apex of the pleura.

Labels (Fig. 2):
R. BRACHIOCEPHALIC V.
PHRENIC N.
INT. THOR. A. & V.
BRACHIOCEPHALIC A.
SCAL. ANT. M.
TRACHEA
ANSA SUBCLAVIA
VAGUS N.
REC. LARYNG. N.
SUBCLAV. A.
ESOPH.
COSTOCERV. TRUNK
STELLATE GANG.
HIGHEST INTERCOSTAL A.
8th CERV. N.
1st THOR. N.
2nd INTERCOSTAL N.

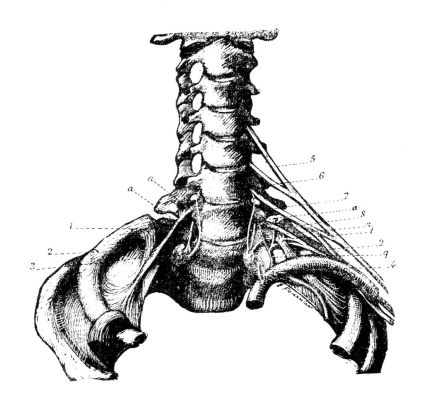

FIG. 3
The suprapleural membrane (Sibson's fascia). (From Sébileau, 1891.) On the right the membrane is intact. On the left, relations of the membrane are shown.

the same relationship to the pleura as the endoabdominal fascia bears to the peritoneum. The endothoracic fascia is a complete connective tissue membrane lining the bones and muscles of the walls of the thorax.

The cleavage plane between the endothoracic fascia and the pleura can readily be exploited for extrapleural procedures such as extrapleural pneumothorax (see Horsley and Bigger, 1953), pneumonectomy, and mediastinal drainage (see Fig. 20), or for extrapleural approaches to the esophagus (see Fig. 131), great vessels (see Fig. 26), or sympathetic trunks (see Fig. 14).

Generally the endothoracic fascia is thin, especially over the mediastinum. The apical part, or suprapleural membrane, is relatively heavy and firmly attached to the first rib and to the seventh cervical and first thoracic vertebrae. It blends medially with the lax connective tissue about the midline viscera. The membrane sends prolongations to the sheaths of the vessels and nerves that pass out of the thorax; these are best appreciated when one is performing extrafascial apicolysis (see Fig. 9).

REMOVAL OF THE FIRST RIB FOR RELIEF OF NEUROVASCULAR COMPRESSION

The removal of an anomalous first rib has long been practiced. Roos (1966) suggested that removal of a normal first rib will relieve neurovascular compression of whatever origin, by allowing the subclavian artery and brachial plexus a roomy exit from the thorax. He advised removal of the rib through the axilla (Fig. 4). In this procedure the arm is raised above the head, tending to lift the neurovascular structures away from the rib. The pectoralis minor muscle arches across the rib and its related structures, and must be divided (Fig. 4 A).

Not shown in Figure 4 A is the clavipectoral fascia (Fig. 5), which encloses the pectoralis minor muscle and must be divided with it. After the pectoralis minor muscle is divided (Fig. 4 B) the operator will come upon the subclavius muscle; however the subclavius muscle, although easily palpable, will not be visible until the heavy upper part (the costo-coracoid membrane) of the clavipectoral fascia which

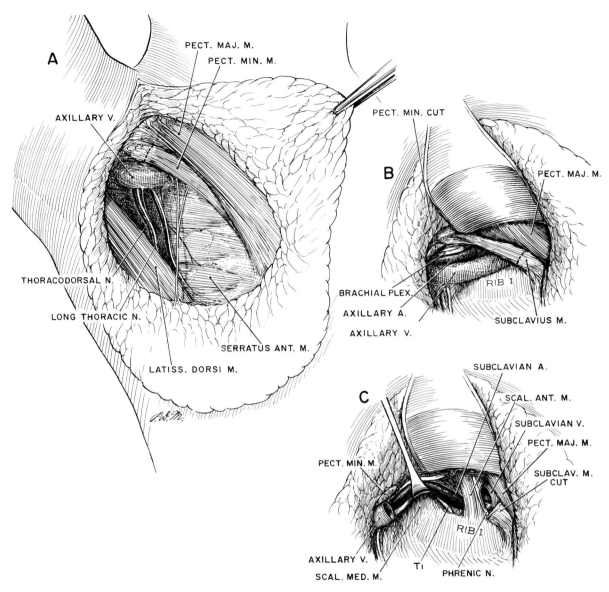

FIG. 4
Removal of the first rib through the axilla.

encloses it is divided. The subclavian vein can now retreat above the rib. Division of the scalenus anterior muscle (sparing the phrenic nerve) allows retraction of the subclavian artery and the lower trunk of the brachial plexus. The rib may now be removed.

Proponents of this approach state that the stellate ganglion or a cervical rib can also be removed through the same route. The ganglion is available after the suprapleural membrane is pushed away, but the view is quite restricted, and

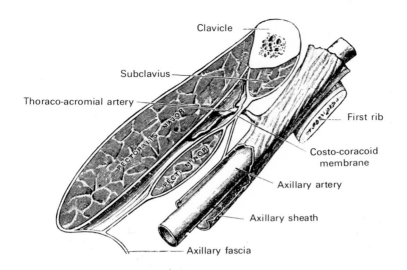

Clavicle

Subclavius

Thoraco-acromial artery

First rib

Costo-coracoid membrane

Axillary artery

Axillary sheath

Axillary fascia

FIG. 5
Fasciae enclosing the pectoral and subclavius muscles. The fascia extending from the pectoralis minor to the clavicle is termed the clavipectoral fascia; its upper thick portion which divides to enclose the subclavius muscle is the costo-coracoid membrane. (From Robinson, 1921.)

sympathectomy is probably better performed by either a transthoracic or a supraclavicular scalene approach. The supraclavicular scalene approach also allows a better assessment of the cause of neurovascular compression and affords a better path for removal of a cervical rib (Edwards, 1962). Removal of the first thoracic rib is, however, more difficult through the scalene approach because the neurovascular structures must be retracted.

A posterior or parascapular approach to the first thoracic rib or to a cervical rib is achieved through an incision which is essentially the same as that used for apical thoracoplasty (see Chapter 2). Such an approach has the disadvantage of not-allowing as good a view of the anterior end of a cervical rib, which is the site of mischief occasioned by such a structure. Brodsky and Gol (1970) have used an anterior infraclavicular approach for removal of the medial part of the first rib. The pectoralis major muscle is split, and the rib is removed subperiosteally, while the neurovascular bundle is retracted laterally and upward.

Mention should also be made of the possibility of removing the first rib from within the thorax. This may be done for distal control of the subclavian artery while the vessels are being exposed during thoracotomy (Mansberger and Linberg, 1965).

REFERENCES

Brodsky, A. E., and Gol, A.: Costoclavicular syndrome. Relief by infraclavicular removal of first rib. South. Med. J. 63:50–58, 1970.

Edwards, E. A.: Anatomic and Clinical Comments on Shoulder Girdle Syndromes. *In* Surgical Treatment of Peripheral Vascular Disease, Barker, W. F., Ed. New York, McGraw-Hill, Blakiston Division, 1962.

Horsley, G. W., and Bigger, I. A.: Operative Surgery, 6th ed. Vol. 1. St. Louis, Mosby, 1953.

Mansberger, A. R., Jr., and Linberg, E. J.: First rib resection for distal exposure of subclavian vessels. Surg. Gynec. Obstet. 120:578–579, 1965.

Robinson, A., Ed.: Cunningham's Manual of Practical Anatomy, 7th ed., Vol. 1. New York, William Wood, 1921.

Roos, D. B.: Transaxillary approach for first rib resection to relieve thoracic outlet syndrome. Ann. Surg. 163:354–358, 1966.

Sébileau, P.: L'appareil suspenseur de la plèvre. Bull. Soc. Anat. Paris 66:410–445, 1891.

THORACIC WALL

POSTEROLATERAL THORACOPLASTY

The aim of thoracoplasty is collapse of the underlying lung by removal of ribs and of the transverse processes of the vertebrae, usually the upper seven. The exposure shown in Figure 6 is intended to emphasize how the upper part of the procedure may be utilized to expose the pedicle of the upper extremity, as for removal of the first rib for relief of neurovascular compression, or as an early step in inter-scapulothoracic amputation. A similar approach limited to the upper intercostal area, often by muscle splitting, can give access for an upper thoracic extrapleural sympathectomy.

The operation of thoracoplasty is well described by Coleman (1953). The incision passes through all but the upper part of the trapezius muscle, a bit of the upper latissimus dorsi, and both rhomboid muscles, allowing the scapula to be retracted away from the ribs and putting the serratus anterior muscle on the stretch. Figure 6 B shows this stage of the procedure with the levator scapulae and most of the trapezius muscle divided, as would be done in the wider exposure used for an amputation.

Placing the incision close to the spine minimizes injury to the nerves and vessels which course close to the vertebral border of the scapula (Fig. 7): the accessory nerve and as-cending branch of the transverse cervical artery beneath the

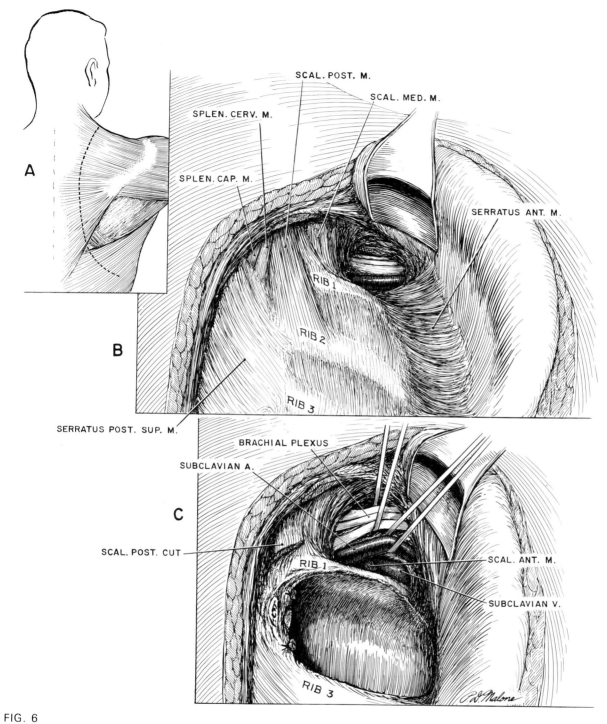

SCAL. POST. M.

SCAL. MED. M.

SPLEN. CERV. M.

SPLEN. CAP. M.

SERRATUS ANT. M.

A

B

RIB 1

RIB 2

RIB 3

SERRATUS POST. SUP. M.

BRACHIAL PLEXUS

SUBCLAVIAN A.

C

SCAL. POST. CUT

SCAL. ANT. M.

RIB 1

SUBCLAVIAN V.

RIB 3

P.D. Malone

FIG. 6

Posterolateral thoracoplasty. A. Line of incision in superficial muscles. B. Parascapular muscles divided and scapula retracted. C. Neurovascular relationships above first rib; second rib is removed for access to first rib.

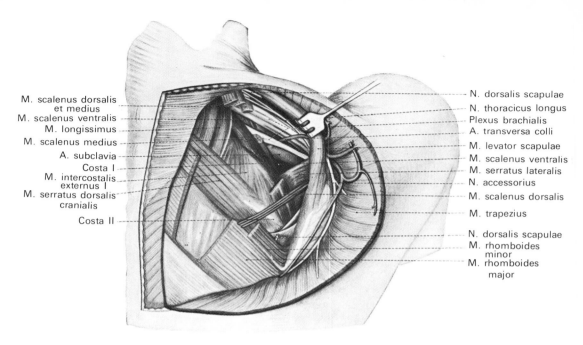

M. scalenus dorsalis et medius
M. scalenus ventralis
M. longissimus
M. scalenus medius
A. subclavia
Costa I
M. intercostalis externus I
M. serratus dorsalis cranialis
Costa II

N. dorsalis scapulae
N. thoracicus longus
Plexus brachialis
A. transversa colli
M. levator scapulae
M. scalenus ventralis
M. serratus lateralis
N. accessorius
M. scalenus dorsalis
M. trapezius
N. dorsalis scapulae
M. rhomboides minor
M. rhomboides major

FIG. 7
Deep upper parascapular structures. (From Hafferl, 1953.)

trapezius muscle, and the dorsal scapular nerve and descending branch of the transverse cervical artery beneath the levator scapulae and rhomboid muscles.

The upper four digitations of the serratus anterior muscle are detached. Division of the insertion of the serratus posterior superior brings the erector spinae muscle into view, and its lateral (iliocostalis) digitations are detached from the ribs, so that this muscle can be retracted medially. When division of the muscle has not been carried quite as high as is shown in Figure 6 B, the second rib is apparently the highest. The safest exposure of the first rib is usually gained by preliminary removal of the second. The insertions of the scalenus muscles will be severed from the first two ribs.

Removal of the first three ribs usually includes their costal cartilages. Progressively smaller amounts of the anterior portions of the ribs below are removed. Posteriorly the entire transverse process of each vertebra is removed with the adjacent head and neck of the rib, except for the transverse process of the first thoracic vertebra, which is only partially removed in order to avoid injury to the eighth cervical and first thoracic roots of the inferior trunk of the brachial plexus

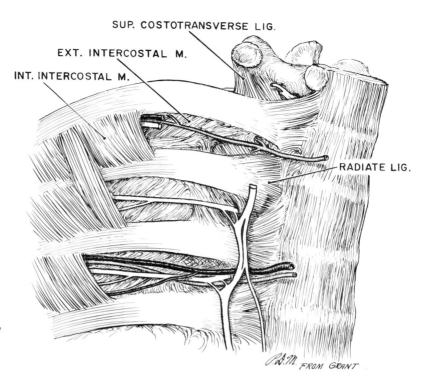

SUP. COSTOTRANSVERSE LIG.

EXT. INTERCOSTAL M.

INT. INTERCOSTAL M.

RADIATE LIG.

FROM GRANT

FIG. 8
Costovertebral junctions and related anterior structures. (After Grant, 1956.)

(see Figs. 1 and 2). The costotransverse and costovertebral (radiate) ligaments will be divided in this step (Fig. 8).

The relationship of intercostal nerves and vessels, and of the sympathetic trunk, to the heads of the ribs must be borne in mind (Fig. 8). At the first rib the brachial plexus, subclavian artery and vein, and the internal thoracic vessels must be avoided.

EXTRAFASCIAL APICOLYSIS

The operation of extrafascial apicolysis (Fig. 9) was described by Semb (1935) as a supplement to apical thoracoplasty. By downward displacement of the apex of the lung it adds a vertical element to the circumferential collapse of the lung. The suprapleural membrane is detached from the first rib, then displaced downward as its prolongations to the brachial plexus and subclavian vessels are divided (Fig. 9). The periosteum and intercostal structures are allowed to remain on the outside of the fascia. Rib regeneration maintains collapse of the lung.

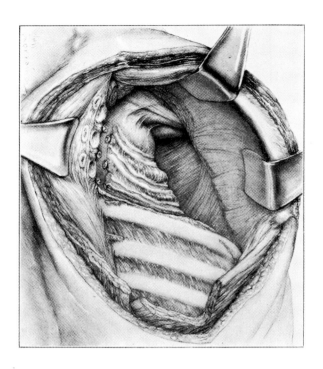

FIG. 9
Extrafascial apicolysis. (From Coleman, 1953.)

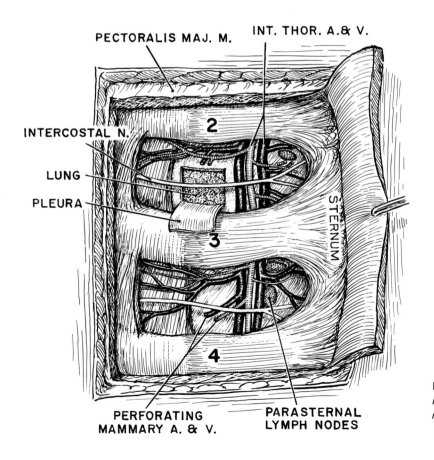

PECTORALIS MAJ. M.

INT. THOR. A.& V.

INTERCOSTAL N.

LUNG

PLEURA

2

3

4

STERNUM

PERFORATING
MAMMARY A. & V.

PARASTERNAL
LYMPH NODES

FIG. 10
Internal thoracic vessels and lymph nodes. (After Testut and Jacob, 1914.)

REMOVAL OF INTERNAL THORACIC LYMPH NODES

The internal thoracic (internal mammary) arteries and lymphatic vessels send perforating branches to the pectoralis major muscle and the breast. These are usually largest in the second and third intercostal spaces. These perforating vessels are divided in radical mastectomy, beneath the muscle origin. The proximity of the pleura (Fig. 10) invites pneumothorax if a retracting vessel stump is sought in the intercostal space.

The internal thoracic lymph nodes may be biopsied by removing the second or third costal cartilage. The operation may be 'extended' to remove the nodes and adjacent pleura (Fig. 11).

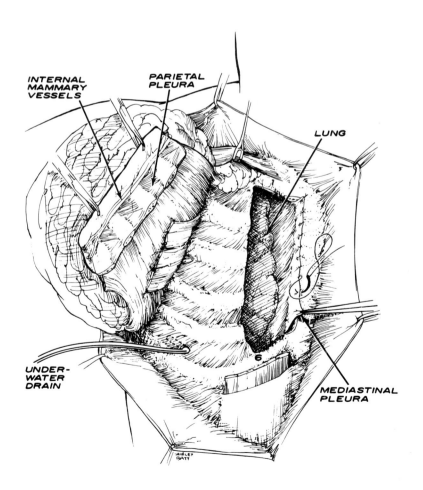

FIG. 11
Removal of sternocostal flap and internal thoracic lymph nodes in extended radical mastectomy. (From Urban, in Cooper, 1971.)

2

SYMPATHECTOMY

Cervicothoracic Sympathectomy

Sympathetic outflow from the spinal cord takes place only through fibers of the thoracic and the upper two lumbar spinal nerves. The surgeon is thus attracted to the thoracic region, since sympathetic denervation of much of the body may be produced by removal of parts or all of the thoracic trunk, and total denervation is effected if the ablation is extended through or below the diaphragm to include the upper lumbar sympathetic trunk as well.

Excellent exposure of the upper thoracic sympathetic trunk and of the stellate ganglion (for cervicothoracic sympathectomy) is obtained by a high thoracotomy, usually through the second intercostal space in the axilla. The long thoracic nerve must be avoided (see Fig. 4). The sympathetic trunk is readily seen through the posterior parietal pleura and the thin endothoracic fascia.

Henry (1957) suggests an extrapleural dissection after removal of the second rib and costal cartilage. The apical pleura is peeled downward, leaving the nerve trunk covered only by the endothoracic fascia. The removal of the entire stellate ganglion is essential if the upper limb is to be well denervated, and for adequate sensory denervation of the heart (p. 154). Horner's syndrome is produced. The degree of fusion of the first thoracic nerve and the inferior cervical ganglia in the formation of the stellate ganglion varies considerably. A constriction often demarcates these two portions of the stellate ganglion (Moore, 1934).

If the inferior cervical ganglion is left behind Horner's syndrome is usually avoided, but, as noted, the anticipated denervation may be incomplete. Collateral pathways for the sympathetic trunk are described by Kuntz (1949) and Edwards (1951).

Cervicothoracic sympathectomy may also be done by a supraclavicular or scalene approach (Figs. 12 and 13). No important structures are endangered as one successively encounters the platysma, supraclavicular nerves, external jugular vein, and the omohyoid muscle. The underlying internal jugular vein must be avoided when dividing the clavicular head of the sternocleidomastoid muscle. The scalenus

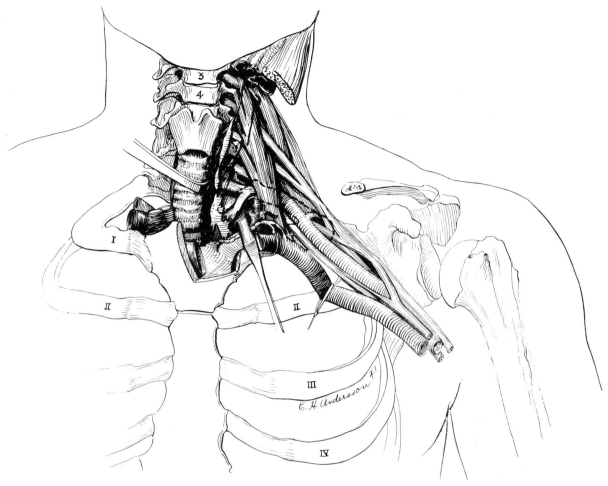

FIG. 12
Stellate ganglion and origin of the brachial plexus. (From Edwards, 1941.)

anterior muscle is exposed after retracting the overlying 'fat pad.' The transverse cervical artery crosses the muscle; the suprascapular artery may also be seen, but it may lie lower under the clavicle. The phrenic nerve, accompanied by the ascending cervical artery, descends beneath the thin scalene fascia. Exceptionally, it is embedded in the muscle.

Division of the scalene muscle exposes the suprapleural membrane. The membrane is separated from the first rib, and the underlying pleura and lung are displaced downward to expose the sympathetic trunk. Many vessels lie in close proximity to the stellate ganglion. These include the deep cervical, highest intercostal, and vertebral arteries, and the vertebral and other veins (see Figs. 1 and 2). The advantage of this exposure lies in the opportunity for simultaneous exploration for causes of neurovascular compression, such

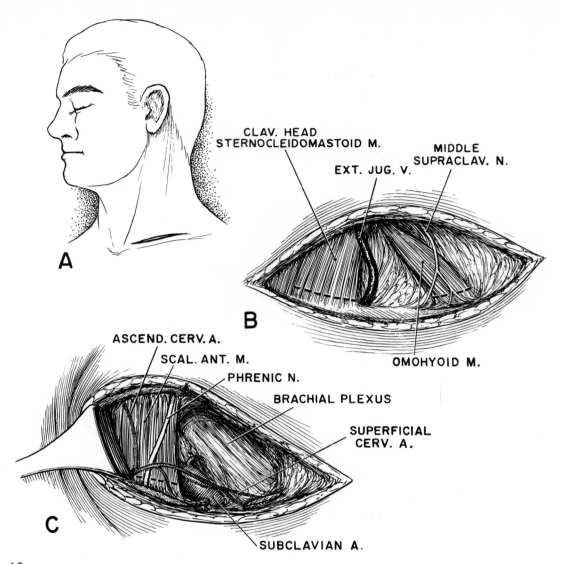

FIG. 13

Supraclavicular (scalene) approach for cervicothoracic sympathectomy. The line of section of the sternocleido-mastoid and omohyoid muscles is indicated in B, and of the scalenus anterior muscle in C.

as a cervical rib. Disadvantages are the narrowness and depth of the exposure.

The once-popular posterior extrapleural approach for cervicothoracic sympathectomy is well illustrated by Homans (1939) and Henry (1957). This approach (see Fig. 26) was based on the presumed necessity for preganglionic section (the stellate ganglion was not removed), and for ablation of the second and third intercostal nerves (to prevent regeneration). The exposure was centered on the third rib. The trapezius was here cut across, and the rhomboid and erector

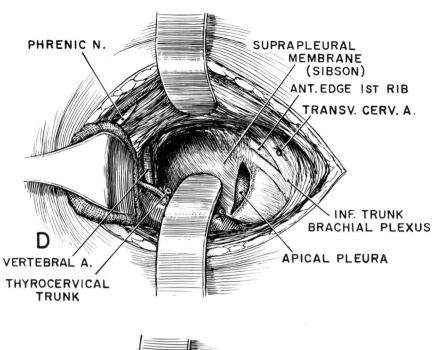

PHRENIC N.
SUPRAPLEURAL MEMBRANE (SIBSON)
ANT. EDGE IST RIB
TRANSV. CERV. A.
INF. TRUNK BRACHIAL PLEXUS
APICAL PLEURA
D
VERTEBRAL A.
THYROCERVICAL TRUNK

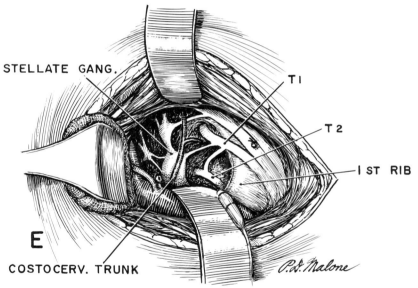

STELLATE GANG.
T1
T2
IST RIB
E
COSTOCERV. TRUNK

P.D. Malone

FIG. 13

Supraclavicular (scalene) approach for cervicothoracic sympathectomy (continued). D. Incision of the suprapleural membrane (Sibson's fascia). E. Exposure of the stellate ganglion. The sponge and anterior retractor protect the internal jugular vein and phrenic nerve.

spinae muscles were split. The posterior part of the third rib and the transverse process of the third vertebra were removed and the pleura was pushed away. According to Henry, the origins of the intercostal nerves are more easily exposed through the anterior approach offered by a thoracotomy.

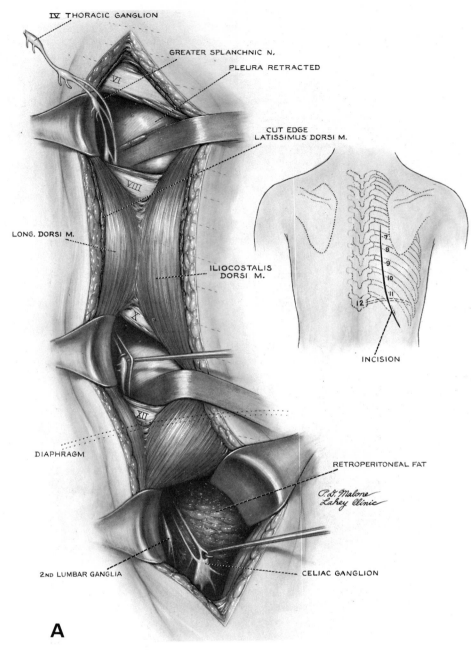

IV THORACIC GANGLION

GREATER SPLANCHNIC N.

PLEURA RETRACTED

CUT EDGE LATISSIMUS DORSI M.

LONG. DORSI M.

ILIOCOSTALIS DORSI M.

INCISION

DIAPHRAGM

RETROPERITONEAL FAT

P. d. Malone
Lahey Clinic

2ND LUMBAR GANGLIA

CELIAC GANGLION

A

FIG. 14

Transthoracic and subdiaphragmatic extrapleural sympathectomy and splanchnicectomy. A. The surgical approach. B. Scope of the sympathectomy (on facing page). (From Poppen, 1947.)

Thoracolumbar Sympathectomy

Thoracolumbar sympathectomy was the culmination of efforts to achieve greater and greater denervation in the treatment of hypertension. Surgical intervention ranged from the adrenal denervation of Crile, to the supradiaphragmatic

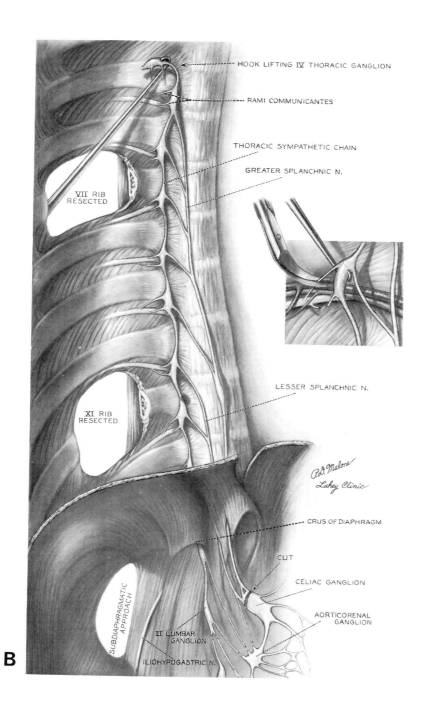

HOOK LIFTING IV THORACIC GANGLION

RAMI COMMUNICANTES

THORACIC SYMPATHETIC CHAIN

GREATER SPLANCHNIC N.

VII RIB RESECTED

LESSER SPLANCHNIC N.

XI RIB RESECTED

R.S. Malone
Lahey Clinic

CRUS OF DIAPHRAGM

CUT

CELIAC GANGLION

AORTICORENAL GANGLION

SUBDIAPHRAGMATIC APPROACH

II LUMBAR GANGLION

ILIOHYPOGASTRIC N.

B

extrapleural splanchnicectomy of Peet, to the combined supra- and infradiaphragmatic sympathectomy and splanchnicectomy of Smithwick (in Cole, 1956). Thoracolumbar sympathectomy is well described by Poppen (1947) (Fig. 14). The lower end of the incision offers a view of the adrenal (suprarenal) gland and kidney, an advantage when biopsy of those organs is desired.

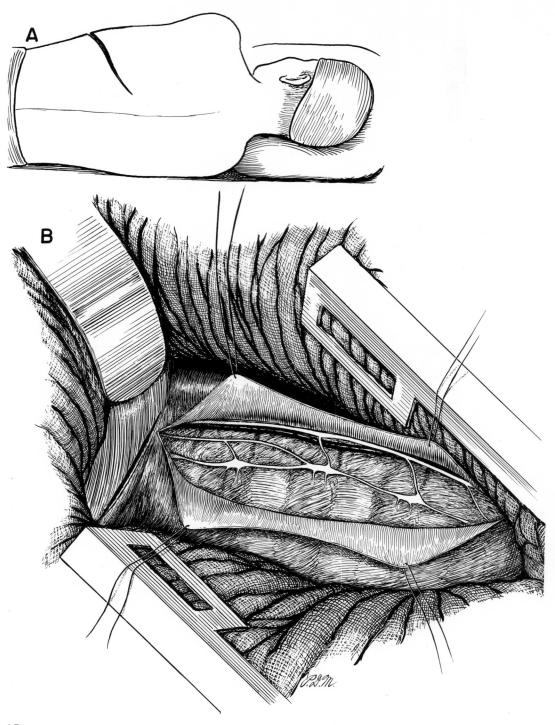

FIG. 15
Transthoracic and transdiaphragmatic sympathectomy and splanchnicectomy. A. The thoractomy incision. B. The sympathetic trunk and splanchnic nerve dissected through the pleura. The diaphragm is incised.

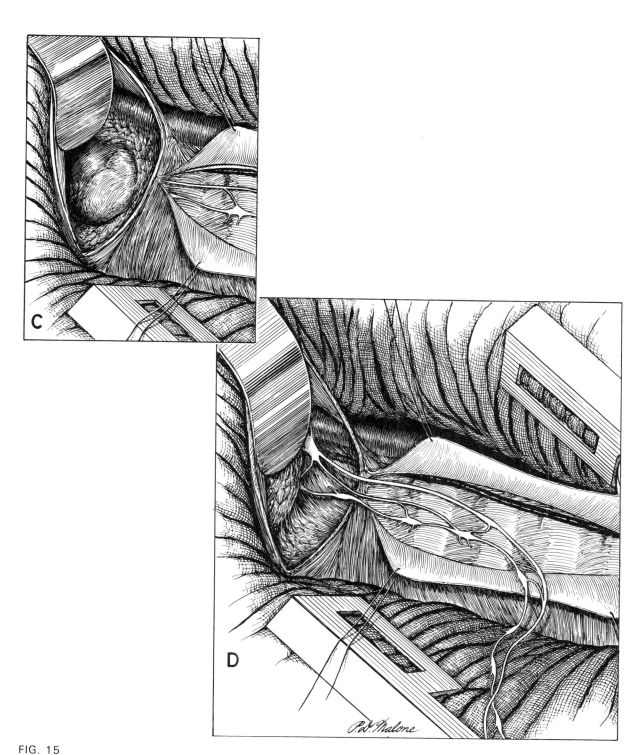

FIG. 15
Transthoracic and transdiaphragmatic sympathectomy and splanchnicectomy (continued). *C. The kidney and adrenal, seen through the renal fascia, are available for biopsy. They are retracted in D, and the infradiaphragmatic dissection is completed. (After Linton* et al., *1947.)*

Grimson (1941) performed a transpleural operation through the beds of the third and the tenth rib, removing the entire thoracic chain. By following the splanchnic nerves through the diaphragm he was able to bring up and remove the celiac ganglion. He had variable success in obtaining portions of the lumbar chain by following the thoracic trunk.

Linton *et al.* (1947), by making a 'generous incision' through the bed of the ninth rib and opening the diaphragm 'widely' in front of the twelfth rib, obtained a better view of the retroperitoneum, permitting removal of two or three lumbar segments of the sympathetic trunk and exploration of the kidney and the adrenal gland (Fig. 15).

REFERENCES

Cole, W. H., Ed.: Operative Technic in Specialty Surgery, 2nd ed. New York, Appleton-Century-Crofts, 1956.

Coleman, F. P.: Surgery for Pulmonary Tuberculosis. Chapter 35 *in* Operative Surgery, 6th ed., Horsley, G. W., and Bigger, I. A., Eds. Vol. 1. St. Louis, Mosby, 1953.

Edwards, E. A.: Nonarterial disorders simulating disease of the peripheral arteries. New Eng. J. Med. 225:91–101, 1941.

Edwards, E. A.: Operative anatomy of the lumbar sympathetic chain. Angiology 2:184–198, 1951.

Grant, J. C. B.: An Atlas of Anatomy, 4th ed. Baltimore, Williams & Wilkins, 1956.

Grimson, K. S.: Total thoracic and partial to total lumbar sympathectomy and celiac ganglionectomy in the treatment of hypertension. Ann. Surg. 114:753–775, 1941.

Hafferl, A.: Lehrbuch der topographischen Anatomie. Berlin, Springer, 1953.

Henry, A. K.: Extensile Exposure, 2nd ed. Edinburgh, Livingstone, 1957.

Homans, J.: Circulatory Diseases of the Extremities. New York, Macmillan, 1939.

Horsley, G. W., and Bigger, I. A.: Operative Surgery, 6th ed. Vol. I. St. Louis, Mosby, 1953.

Kuntz, A.: The Neuroanatomic Basis of Surgery of the Autonomic Nervous System. Springfield, Charles C Thomas, 1949.

Linton, R. R., Moore, F. D., Simeone, F. A., Welch, C. E., and White, J. C.: Thoracolumbar sympathectomy for hypertension. Improvements in paravertebral and transpleural routes to facilitate extensive neurectomy. Surg. Clin. N. Amer. 22:1178–1187, 1947.

Moore, D. C.: Stellate Ganglion Block. Techniques—Indications—Uses. Springfield, Charles C Thomas, 1954.

Poppen, J. L.: Extensive combined thoracolumbar sympathectomy in hypertension. Surg. Gynec. Obstet. 84:1117–1123, 1947.

Semb, C.: Thoracoplasty with extrafascial apicolysis. Acta Chir. Scand., vol. 76, Suppl. 37, Part II, 1935.

Testut, J. L., and Jacob, O.: Traité d'anatomie topographique avec applications medico-chirurgicales. Vol. I. Paris, Doin, 1914.

Urban, J. A.: Carcinoma of the Breast. Chapter 20 *in* The Craft of Surgery, Cooper, P., Ed., 2nd ed. Vol. 1. Boston, Little, Brown, 1971.

SECTION 2

The Mediastinum Exclusive of the Heart and Pericardium

THE MEDIASTINUM

BOUNDARIES AND CONTENTS

The mediastinum is that region of the thorax lying between the two pleurae. It is divided into the superior and the inferior mediastinum by a line extending between the junction of the manubrium and the body of the sternum to the lower part of the fourth thoracic vertebra. In the upright position the lower limit of the superior mediastinum descends to the sixth or seventh thoracic vertebra. Within the superior mediastinum lie the tracheal bifurcation, the aortic arch and its branches, and the great veins, including the arch of the azygos vein (Figs. 16, 17, 18). The bifurcation of the pulmonary artery lies at the lower limit of this region or a little below.

The inferior mediastinum is divided into the anterior, middle, and posterior mediastina, the middle mediastinum containing the heart and proximal portions of the great vessels. The thymus lies in the superior and the anterior mediastinum; the root of the lung and descending aorta lie in the posterior mediastinum. The esophagus, vagus nerves, and thoracic duct lie in both the superior and the posterior mediastinum.

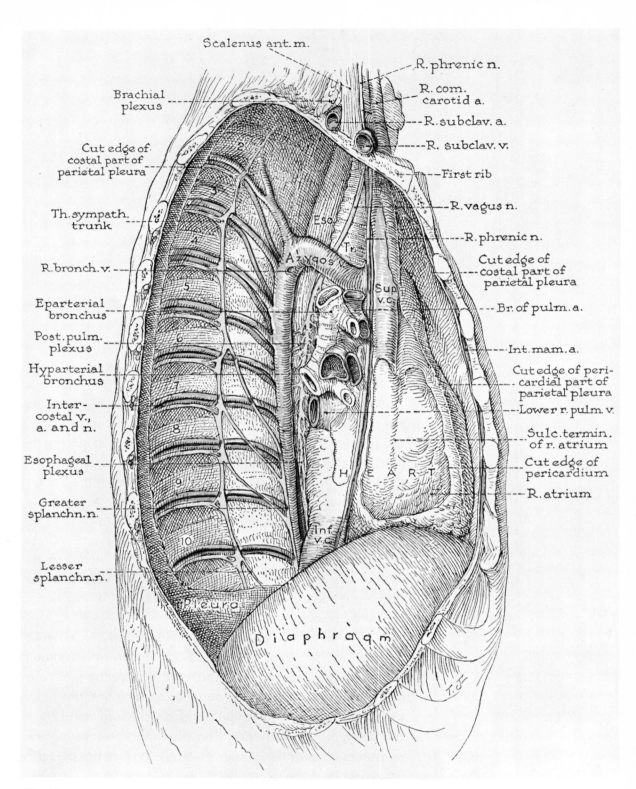

FIG. 16
Right view of mediastinum and root of the lung. (From Jones and Shepard, 1945.)

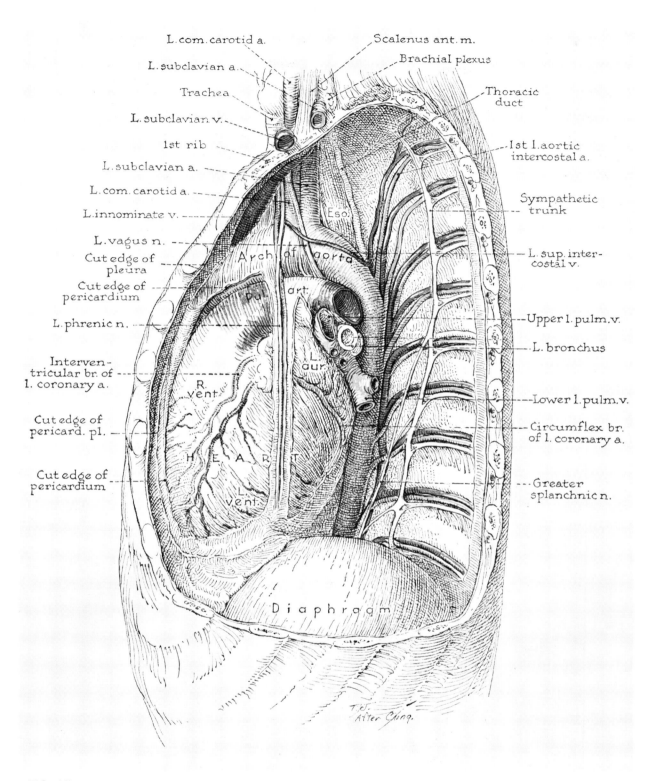

L.com.carotid a.
Scalenus ant.m.
L.subclavian a.
Brachial plexus
Trachea
Thoracic duct
L.subclavian v.
1st rib
1st l.aortic intercostal a.
L.subclavian a.
L.com.carotid a.
Sympathetic trunk
L.innominate v.
L.vagus n.
Cut edge of pleura
L. sup. intercostal v.
Cut edge of pericardium
L.phrenic n.
Upper l.pulm.v.
L. bronchus
Interventricular br. of l. coronary a.
Lower l.pulm.v.
Cut edge of pericard. pl.
Circumflex br. of l. coronary a.
Cut edge of pericardium
Greater splanchnic n.

Eso.
Arch of aorta
Pul. art.
L. aur.
R. vent.
HEART
L. vent.
Diaphragm

T.C.
After Ching.

FIG. 17
Left view of mediastinum and root of the lung. (From Jones and Shepard, 1945.)

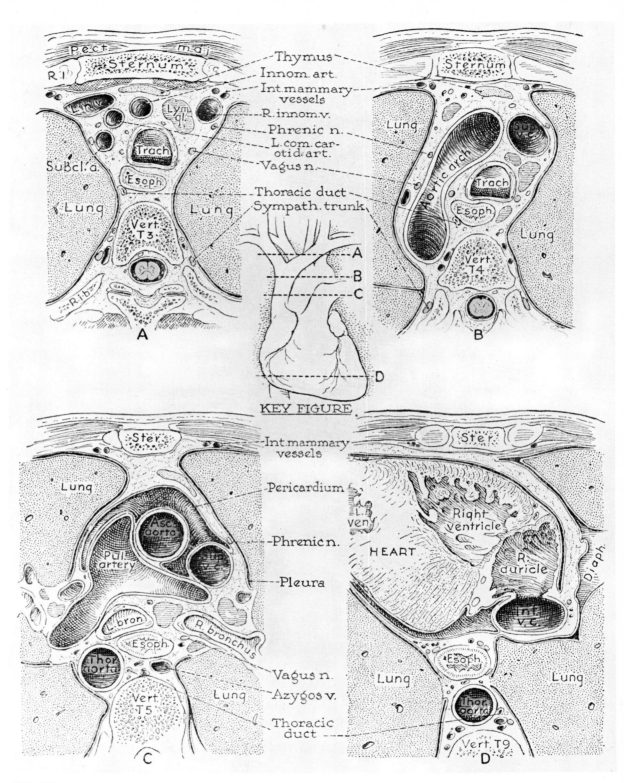

FIG. 18
Cross sections of mediastinum, made at levels indicated by lines designated by corresponding letters in the key figure. The sections are viewed from above. (From Jones and Shepard, 1945.)

MEDIASTINOTOMY AND MEDIASTINOSCOPY

The widest entrance to the superior and the anterior mediastinum is gained by the mid-sternal approach (see Fig. 56). Chapter 5 describes how this approach may be modified and extended to follow these structures. A more limited approach, as for removal of parasternal lymph nodes for biopsy or in extended breast surgery, may be obtained by resection of one or more costal cartilages (see Fig. 11).

Access to the tracheobronchial nodes can be effected by removal of the right second costal cartilage, with lateral retraction of the pleura (McNeill and Chamberlain, 1966) (see Fig. 22). Lung tissue can be removed for biopsy if desired. On the left side the depth of dissection is somewhat limited by the aortic arch.

Because of the downward slope of the upper ribs, much of the superior mediastinum is approachable from the lower neck. Superior-posterior mediastinitis, arising from infection of the retrovisceral space anterior to the cervical prevertebral fascia, can thus be drained down to about the level of the fourth thoracic vertebra by an incision anterior to the lower portion of the sternocleidomastoid muscle (Fig. 19). The lower posterior mediastinum can be entered by posterior rib resection for drainage with or without opening the pleura (Fig. 20), or for extrapleural approaches to structures such as the esophagus (see Fig. 131) or the sympathetic nerves (see Fig. 14).

The 'scalene fat pad' lying in front of the lower part of the scalenus anterior muscle contains internal jugular nodes which possess communications with bronchomediastinal nodes. Biopsy of these nodes, proposed by Daniels (1949), has been useful in the diagnosis of intrathoracic disease. Rouvière (1932) had indicated that the right scalene nodes receive lymphatics from the left lower lobe as well as from all parts of the right lung (see Fig. 98). Experience with cancer of the lung indicates that crossover may occur to either side (Yee *et al.,* 1969). The possibility that scalene-node biopsy may be useful in abdominal disease is suggested by the finding of frequent metastases in left supra-clavicular nodes when intra-abdominal cancer has reached the thoracic duct (Young, 1956).

The prescalene fat pad is approached by a supraclavicular

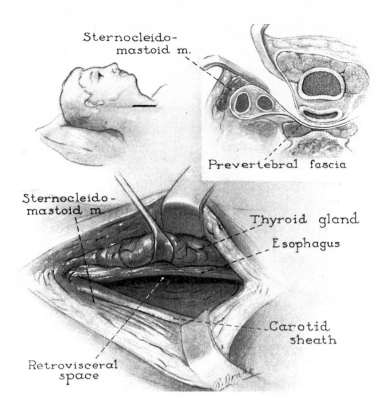

Sternocleido-
mastoid m.

Prevertebral fascia

Sternocleido-
mastoid m.

Thyroid gland

Esophagus

Carotid
sheath

Retrovisceral
space

FIG. 19
*Extrapleural drainage of the superior
mediastinum by cervical mediastinotomy. (From Seybold et al., 1950.)*

incision with or without division of some of the sternocleidomastoid muscle (Paulson, 1967; Watson, 1968) (see Fig.
13). The two heads of that muscle may be split, if care is
taken to avoid the internal jugular vein which lies immediately behind. The pad lies anterior to the thin scalene fascia
which usually protects the phrenic nerve. The dissection
extends medially to the internal jugular vein, above to the
omohyoid muscle, and below to the subclavian vein. In the
field lie varying portions of the external and anterior jugular
veins, branches of the thyrocervical arterial trunk, and lymph
trunks, including the thoracic duct on the left side (see Figs.
12 and 133). The hazards caused by the proximity of other
structures are emphasized by the occasional complications
of lymph fistula, air embolism, and Horner's syndrome
(Skinner, 1963).

A superior sulcus tumor can be approached for biopsy
directly through the scalene area after division of the scalenus anterior muscle and displacement of the suprapleural
membrane from the first rib (McGoon, 1964). The exposure
is similar to that obtained by the scalene approach for cervicothoracic sympathectomy (see Figs. 12 and 13).

Extensions of the scalene fat biopsy have led to more direct cervicomediastinal exploration. Harken and associates (1954) first did this from the scalene area, by passing a finger, then a lighted laryngoscope, beneath the carotid sheath and down the anterolateral aspect of the trachea to the principal bronchus. Pretracheal and paratracheal nodes can thus be removed for biopsy. On the left side the arch of the aorta may be difficult to displace for the lowest nodes. Dissection can be carried to the carotid sheath, or behind the sternum. Injury may occur to the subclavian, internal jugular, or brachiocephalic vein, the pleura, and on the left to the thoracic duct.

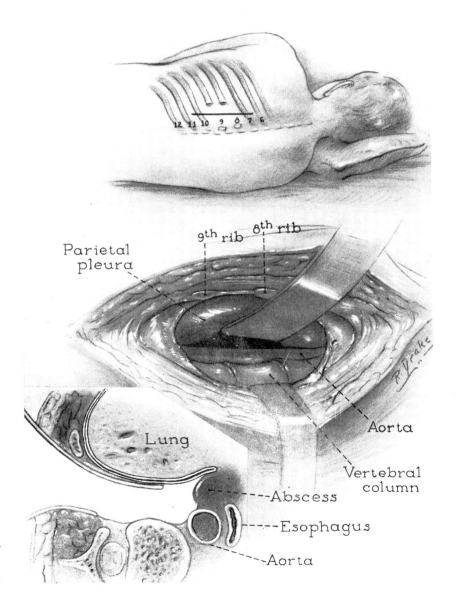

FIG. 20
Extrapleural drainage of the posterior mediastinum by posterior mediastinotomy. (From Seybold et al., 1950.)

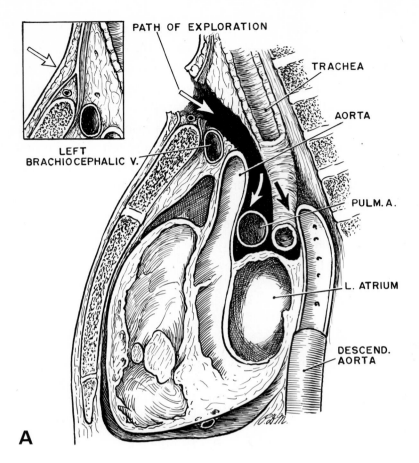

PATH OF EXPLORATION

TRACHEA

AORTA

LEFT
BRACHIOCEPHALIC V.

PULM. A.

L. ATRIUM

DESCEND.
AORTA

A

FIG. 21

Cervicomediastinal exploration by suprasternal route. A. Path of exploration. B. Procedure, and relationships encountered at mediastinoscopy. (a) Infiltration of local anesthetic in suprasternal area; (b) exposure of trachea; (c) relationship of mediastinal structures to exploring finger; (d) relationship of mediastinal structures as encountered through mediastinoscope. (B is from Morton and Guinn, 1971.)

More recently cervicomediastinal exploration has been carried out through a suprasternal incision (Carlens, 1959). Although it does not expose the scalene area, this operation gives more direct access to the pretracheal and paratracheal nodes of both sides, even to the inferior tracheobronchial nodes ('nodes of the carina'). The superior tracheobronchial nodes at the lateral angle of the trachea and bronchus may be seen on the right but are sometimes difficult to approach behind the aortic arch on the left. The suprasternal incision is similar to but lower than that for tracheostomy (Fig. 21). It passes through the suprasternal space which lies between the superficial or enveloping layer of deep fascia and the infrahyoid fascia which encloses the infrahyoid muscles. The space contains fat and the anterior jugular arch, which may be large. The infrahyoid fascia is opened in its middle, avascular line, the path of exploration now lying in front, or to each side, of the trachea, exterior to the pretracheal fascia. Structures one may encounter an-

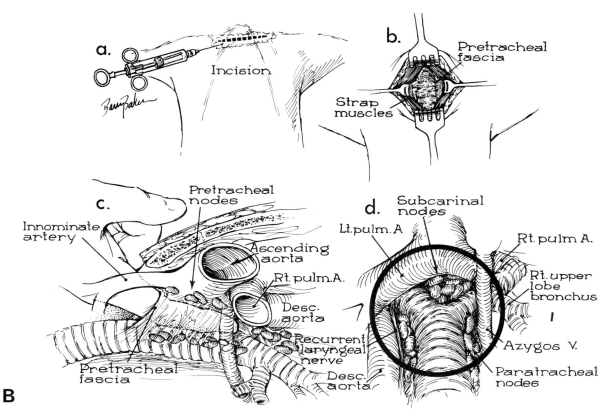

FIG. 21
Cervicomediastinal exploration by suprasternal route. (Continued. See legend on facing page.)

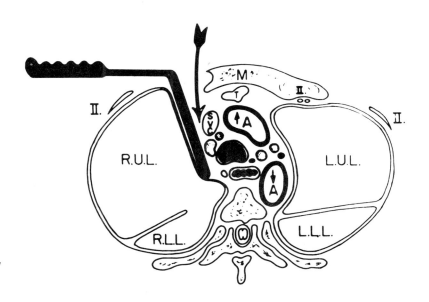

FIG. 22
Mediastinal biopsy via the right second costal cartilage. (From McNeill and Chamberlain, 1966.)

terior to the trachea are inferior thyroid veins, a low-lying thyroid, or the thymus, the first two branches of the aortic arch and rarely the arch itself, a high-lying brachiocephalic vein, and, when present, a thyroidea ima artery. As the mediastinoscope is pushed downward, the presence of the azygos vein, lateral to the right principal bronchus, should be remembered. On the left, the recurrent laryngeal nerve may be encountered at the same level.

By energetic blunt dissection, and using a long mediastinoscope, Specht (1965) has carried the dissection anterior to the great veins into the anterior mediastinum, behind the trachea even to the lower esophagus, to the left of the aortic arch, and to each side of the trachea to the lowermost part of the hilum of the lung on either side. Laterally, the right vagus has been sectioned for pulmonary osteoarthropathy, cysts have been emptied, and paravertebral neurofibromas removed. The risks of such procedures are emphasized by complications observed even in more limited mediastinal explorations. In 6490 cases collected by Ashbaugh (1970), there were 22 instances of injury to a recurrent laryngeal nerve, 3 to the phrenic nerve, 1 to the esophagus, and 1 to a large lymph trunk, in addition to 48 cases of significant hemorrhage and 43 cases of pneumothorax.

References

Ashbaugh, D. G.: Mediastinoscopy. Arch. Surg. 100:568–573, 1970.

Carlens, E.: Mediastinoscopy. A method for inspection and tissue biopsy in the superior mediastinum. Dis. Chest 36:343–352, 1959.

Daniels, A. C.: A method of biopsy useful in diagnosing certain intrathoracic diseases. Dis. Chest 16:360–367, 1949.

Harken, D. E., Black, H., Clauss, R., and Farrand, R. E.: A simple cervicomediastinal exploration for tissue diagnosis of intrathoracic disease. New Eng. J. Med. 251:1041–1044, 1954.

Jones, T., and Shepard, W. C.: A Manual of Surgical Anatomy. Philadelphia, W. B. Saunders, 1945.

McGoon, D. C.: Transcervical technic for removal of specimen from superior sulcus tumor for pathologic study. Ann. Surg. 159:407–410, 1964.

McNeill, T. M., and Chamberlain, J. M.: Diagnostic anterior mediastinotomy. Ann. Thorac. Surg. 2:532–539, 1966.

Morton, J. R., and Guinn, G. A.: Mediastinoscopy using local anesthesia. Amer J. Surg. 122:696–698, 1971.

Paulson, D. L.: Carcinoma of the lung. Current Problems in Surgery, November, 1967.

Rouvière, H.: Anatomie des lymphatiques de l'homme. Paris, Masson, 1932.

Seybold, W. D., Johnson, M. A., III, and Leary, W. V.: Perforation of the esophagus. An analysis of 50 cases and an account of experimental studies. Surg. Clin. N. Amer. 30:1155–1183, 1950.

Skinner, D. B.: Scalene-lymph-node biopsy. Reappraisal of risks and indications. New Eng. J. Med. 268:1324–1329, 1963.

Specht, G.: Erweiterte Mediastinoskopie. Thoraxchirurgie 13: 401–407, 1965.

Watson, W. L., Ed.: Lung Cancer. A Study of Five Thousand Memorial Hospital Cases. St. Louis, Mosby, 1968.

Yee, J., Llewellyn, G. A., Williams, P. A., May, I. A., and Dugan, D. J.: Scalene lymph node dissection. A study of 354 consecutive dissections. Amer. J. Surg. 118:596–601, 1969.

Young, J. M.: The thoracic duct in malignant disease. Amer. J. Path. 32:253–269, 1956.

NORMAl VARiATiONS iN bRANChES
of ThE AORTiC ARCh

PATTERNS OF ORIGIN OF THE
MAJOR ARTERIES

There is considerable variation in the origin of the six major arteries coming from the arch of the aorta, that is, the common carotid, subclavian, and vertebral arteries of each side. A rare seventh branch, the thyroidea ima artery (see Fig. 48), originating from the aortic arch in 0.36 per cent (Hollinshead, 1968), will be considered separately in Chapter 8. Various types of branching of the aortic arch with their frequency are shown in Figure 23.

Robinson (1923) mentions other rare patterns of origin of the arteries, with comparative anatomical notes. The patterns include (1) each of the six arteries (common carotid, subclavian, and vertebral) arising as a separate branch; (2) two stems (a right subclavian and a common trunk for the two carotids and the left subclavian, or two brachiocephalic trunks); and (3) one stem dividing into right and left brachiocephalic trunks. Another unusual pattern, with common origin for both common carotid arteries and the right vertebral artery, is shown in Figure 50.

A right common carotid artery arising as in Figure 23 H, or a left common carotid artery as in Figure 23 D, courses

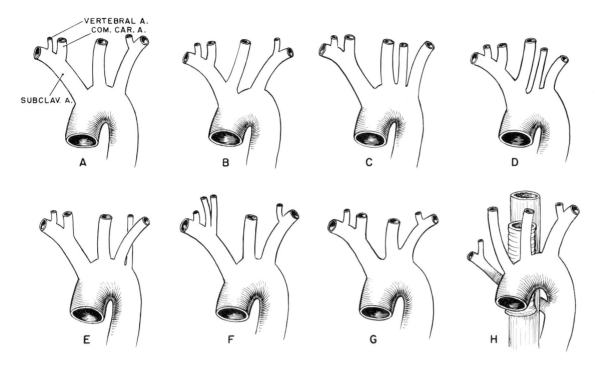

FIG. 23

Variations in origin of vessels arising from the aortic arch. (The percentages represent the frequencies observed in 516 Japanese subjects by Adachi, 1928.) A. The ''normal'' pattern—83%. B. The left common carotid artery arising from the brachiocephalic trunk (innominate artery)—11%. C. The left vertebral artery arising from the aortic arch, between the left common carotid and the left subclavian artery—4%. D. The left common carotid artery arising from the brachiocephalic trunk, with the left vertebral artery arising from the aortic arch—0.6%. E. The left vertebral artery arising as the last branch of the aortic arch—0.6%. F. The right internal and external carotid arteries arising from the brachiocephalic trunk—0.2%. G. Formation of a left brachiocephalic trunk is extremely rare, and was not encountered by Adachi. H. A right retro-esophageal subclavian artery arising as the last branch of the aortic arch—0.2%. Generally, the incidence is thought to be 0.5% (see Chapter 6).

across the trachea, where the arteries are liable to injury in tracheostomy.

VARIATIONS OF ORIGIN OF THE VERTEBRAL ARTERIES

Adachi (1928) found the right and left vertebral arteries arising from the respective subclavian arteries in 95 per cent of 516 cadavers. In the remaining 28 cases the right vertebral artery came from the subclavian, while the left was a branch of the aortic arch, most often arising between the left common carotid artery and the brachiocephalic trunk. The left arose as the last branch of the arch in only three instances. Adachi never encountered a right vertebral artery originating from the arch even in instances of retro-esophageal right subclavian artery. Rarely when there is a retro-esophageal right subclavian artery the right vertebral artery may originate from the common carotid (see Fig. 50). This is discussed in Chapter 8 with reference to the course of the inferior laryngeal nerve. Adachi cites two cases of the right vertebral artery originating from the upper internal carotid, gaining entrance to the skull through the hypoglossal canal in one case and through the transverse foramen of the first cervical vertebra in the other. The origin of a left vertebral artery from the common carotid is 'exceedingly rare.' The site of origin of either vertebral artery from its subclavian parent is usually located quite proximal, opposite the origin of the internal thoracic. Unusually the vertebral artery may originate more distally, sometimes in common with the thyrocervical or the costocervical trunk (Fig. 24).

There may be great variation in size of the two vertebral arteries, one of them contributing almost nothing to the basilar artery. With 'normal origin,' the left is larger than the right in about half of the cases, of equal size in a fourth, and smaller in the remainder. When the left vertebral artery originates from the arch of the aorta, it is usually the smaller vessel (Adachi, 1928).

In 92 per cent of cases in which both vertebral arteries originated from the subclavian arteries, Adachi found the vertebral artery entering the ipsilateral transverse foramen of the sixth cervical vertebra. In the remaining 8 per cent either vertebral artery entered as low as the seventh or as high as the fourth cervical vertebra. In general a low origin, that is the right common from close to the brachiocephalic or the left from the arch, tended to be associated with a greater propensity for entrance in the fourth or fifth cervical vertebra. When a vertebral artery enters high, there is often an additional rudimentary vertebral artery entering the sixth cervical vertebra (Fig. 24 A).

The course of the vertebral artery entering the sixth cervical vertebra lies between the longus colli muscle medially and the scalenus anterior laterally, but the vessel must perforate the longus colli or capitis muscle when it enters at the fourth or fifth cervical vertebra. With an unusual origin or course the vertebral artery may run anterior to the inferior thyroid artery or may give rise to that vessel.

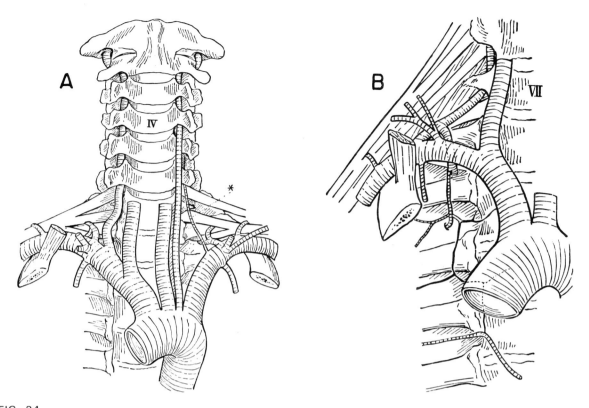

FIG. 24

Variations in origin and course of the vertebral arteries. A. The left vertebral artery shows anomalous origin and course, with a second rudimentary artery of standard pattern. B. The right vertebral artery takes origin in common with the costocervical trunk. (From Adachi, 1928.)

The thoracic duct ordinarily crosses anterior to the left vertebral artery, but origin of the artery from the aortic arch usually brings it medial to the duct. When an accessory rudiment exists, the duct lies anterior to it.

REFERENCES

Adachi, B.: Das Arteriensystem der Japaner. 2 vols. Tokyo, Kenkyusha, 1928.

Edwards, J. E.: Malformations of the aortic arch system manifested as "vascular rings." Lab. Invest. 2:56–75, 1953.

Hollinshead, W. H.: Anatomy for Surgeons, 2nd ed. Vol. 1. New York, Hoeber, 1968.

Robinson, A.: Cunningham's Text-book of Anatomy, 5th ed. New York, William Wood, 1923.

exposures of the aorta and great vessels

THORACIC EXPOSURES

A mid-sternal approach gives optimal exposure for the ascending aorta, the aortic arch, brachiocephalic trunk, the left common carotid artery, and the great veins of the superior mediastinum. The sternum may be split only in its upper extent, but then it must be divided transversely into one of the intercostal spaces, generally the third or fourth of one side or the other. This allows wider retraction and frees the veins from their apical fascial attachment. Although the midline exposure lies between the two pleurae, a transverse extension is easiest transpleurally. Such an extension to the left brings into good view the distal aortic arch with the left subclavian and vertebral arteries.

The main pulmonary artery is accessible from a mid-sternal incision or a left anterolateral thoracotomy. This latter exposure can be extrapleural (Yao and Mustard, 1969). The hila of the lungs are poorly exposed by a mid-sternal approach, but the exposure of a hilum can be improved by extending the incision in the ipsilateral first and sixth intercostal spaces, creating a 'trap door' of that side of the chest wall (Kerr and Warfield, 1928). Deliberate exposure of the right or left main pulmonary artery, as for the Blalock subclavian–pulmonary artery anastomosis (done for palliation of the tetralogy of Fallot), is accomplished by a high antero-lateral thoracotomy (Fig. 25). Most surgeons prefer to use the subclavian artery that arises from the brachiocephalic trunk, because kinking is less likely than when the other subclavian artery is used. Thoracotomy is therefore per-formed on the side opposite the aortic arch. Mobilization of the subclavian artery is begun distally. Proper length requires ligation and division of the thyrocervical trunk, costocervical trunk, vertebral artery, and internal thoracic artery. Division of the pulmonary ligament allows the pulmonary artery to be drawn upward more freely, if that should be necessary.

Some diminution in size of the arm on the side of the subclavian division is often seen, but frank gangrene of the arm has been observed only rarely (Webb and Burford, 1952). Perhaps in such instances there may be anatomic abnormalities of the collateral arterial vessels, although they have not been demonstrated.

Horner's syndrome on the side of the anastomosis has been observed rather often. It is not established whether this is related to damage to the ansa subclavia or to vascular deprivation of the cervical ganglia.

The distal aortic arch and the proximal left subclavian and vertebral arteries are best exposed by a posterolateral thoracotomy in the fourth left intercostal space or the bed of the fifth rib, with division of the adjacent ribs, as used for operation on coarctation of the aorta (see Fig. 35). Expo-sure of the arch and much of the descending aorta, as for aneurysm, is generally obtained by a somewhat lower pos-terolateral incision as through the left fifth intercostal space or rib bed. A limited view of the origin of the left subclavian artery, as for simple ligature, can be obtained extrapleurally from behind by removing the proximal part of the second rib and adjacent transverse process (Henry, 1957) (Fig. 26). A view of the distal portion of the subclavian artery can also be obtained from within the thorax by removing some of the first rib (Mansberger and Linberg, 1965).

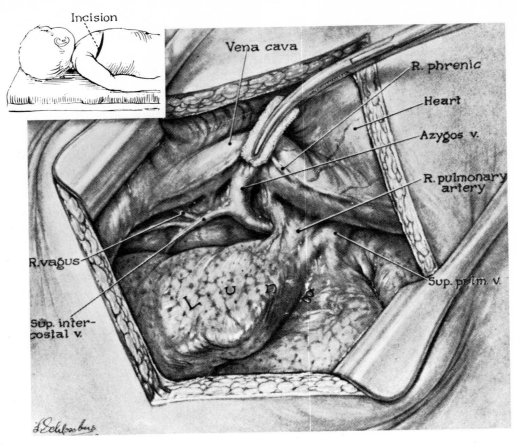

Incision

Vena cava

R. phrenic

Heart

Azygos v.

R. pulmonary artery

R. vagus

Sup. pulm. v.

Sup. intercostal v.

L u n g

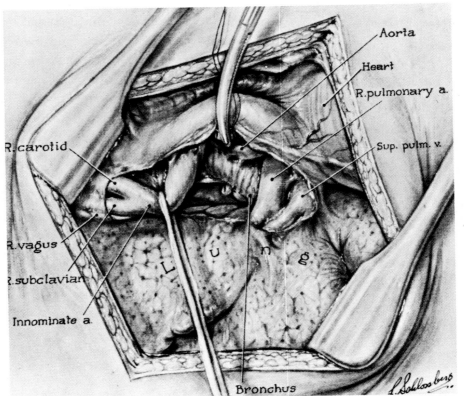

Aorta

Heart

R. pulmonary a.

R. carotid

Sup. pulm. v.

R. vagus

R. subclavian

Innominate a.

L u n g

Bronchus

FIG. 25
Two stages in exposure for subclavian–pulmonary artery anastomosis for tetralogy of Fallot. (From Blalock, 1948.
Blalock entered the pleural cavity through the second or third intercostal space. Others use the fourth.)

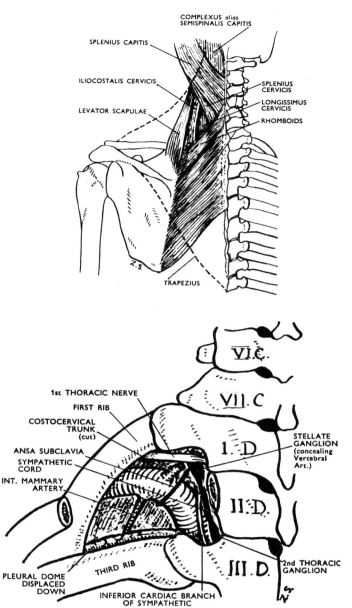

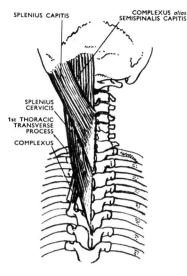

FIG. 26
Extrapleural exposure of the origin of the left subclavian artery and the sympathetic trunk. (From Henry, 1957.) Upper left: Muscle relationships in the area of operation. Upper right: Deeper muscles of the region. Left: Structures seen after removal of portion of the second rib and transverse process of the vertebra.

EXPOSURE EXTENDED TO THE NECK

The simplest extension in this category is that used for midline structures as in a cervicothoracic exposure of the thyroid, parathyroids, or thymus. The usual collar incision is met with a median sternotomy, either full length or limited (see Fig. 46).

Anterolateral structures, such as the contents of the carotid sheath or the vertebral artery, may often be adequately

3

exposed by section of some or all of the sternocleidomastoid, sternohyoid, and sternothyroid muscles with their respective fasciae. A further increase in exposure is gained by excising the medial end of the clavicle alone, or with the adjacent joint and manubrium. Again, such an incision may be connected with a median sternotomy, or extended by sectioning the first two costal cartilages (Amato *et al.,* 1969). Wider exposures, capable of axillary extension, are considered below.

The terminal subclavian and internal jugular veins both lie close to the lateral edge of the sternocleidomastoid muscle. Here the subclavian vein receives the external jugular and anterior jugular veins. This line also marks the lateral edge of the scalenus anterior muscle. In order to avoid injury to these veins, Henry (1957) suggests identifying the finger-tip-sized lateral diverticulum of the suprasternal space, which separates the ensheathed sternocleidomastoid muscle anteriorly from the infrahyoid fascia and muscles posteriorly. The great veins lie behind the infrahyoid fascia.

Several deep tributaries enter the major veins at or near the formation of the brachiocephalic vein. The largest is usually the vertebral. It lies behind the internal jugular and in front of its companion artery (see Fig. 1). It terminates in the uppermost portion of the brachiocephalic vein. The posterior jugular, and, on a deeper plane, the deep cervical vein, also terminating here, start by connecting with the intravertebral plexus at the foramen magnum. They parallel the vertebral vein, the three vessels bearing a reciprocal relationship in size. The major brachiocephalic venous channels, with their tributaries, lie anterior to the major arteries and must be retracted for proper access to the arteries. This often involves division of some veins, with or without re-anastomosis. In general, there is progressively more difficulty with venous return as one ligates at more proximal venous levels (see Fig. 29).

The phrenic nerve usually lies behind the subclavian vein on its way into the chest; exceptionally, it may lie in front of it. The small nerve to the subclavius lies behind the clavicle anterior to the subclavian vein. Frequently, it includes a sizable accessory phrenic component which joins the phrenic nerve immediately below the subclavian vein (see Fig. 1).

CERVICO-AXILLARY EXTENSIONS
OF STERNOTOMY

The major obstacles to a continuous view of the superior mediastinum, base of the neck, and axilla are: the sternum in the thorax, the clavicle with the sternocleidomastoid and subclavius muscles in the neck, and the tendons of the pectoralis major and minor in the axilla. One approach to this extended exposure is that of Killian (1951), who sectioned the manubrium on one or both sides, cut the pectoralis major muscle from the lower clavicle, and retracted the clavicle and manubrium upward (Fig. 27). Sencert (1918) suggested an exposure by creating a claviculo-pectoral or sternoclaviculopectoral pedicle (Fig. 28).

A simpler alternative is to combine the fairly standard cervical incision used in axillary-subclavian exposure, with a mid-sternal incision. The sternoclavicular joint is preserved. A portion of the clavicle is excised (Fig. 29). The cephalic vein, an important collateral trunk, is encountered in the deltopectoral groove arching medially to its termination in the axillary vein deep in the deltopectoral triangle. In removal of the mid-portion of the clavicle, the transverse scapular (suprascapular) vessels are subject to injury. The subclavius muscle is seen covered by the costo-coracoid fascia stretching tautly across the neurovascular structures of the

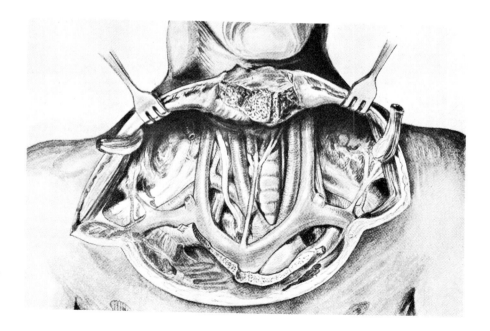

FIG. 27
Cervicothoracic exposure by bilateral sternoclavicular elevation. (From Killian, 1951.)

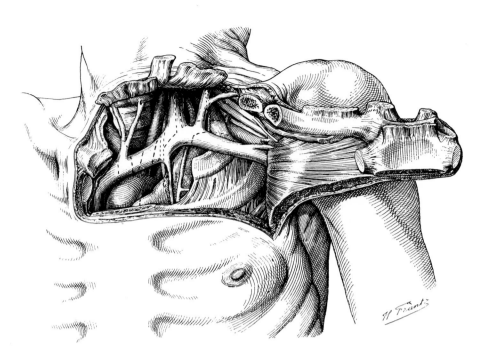

FIG. 28
Cervicothoracic exposure by sterno-clavicular-pectoral pedicle. (From Sencert, 1918.)

upper limb (see Fig. 5). It must be divided. As the lower cervical region is opened by section of the clavicle, the sterno-cleidomastoid and the infrahyoid muscles encased in their fasciae are exposed. On sectioning the infrahyoid fascia and muscles, a view is obtained in continuity of the brachio-cephalic, lower internal jugular, subclavian, and axillary veins. Retraction of these structures downward reveals the scalenus anterior muscle with the phrenic nerve, and branches of the thyrocervical arterial trunk. Upon dividing the scalenus anterior muscle the entire arch of artery to the upper limb and the proximal reaches of the vertebral and carotid vessels are revealed. Laterally, one can display the brachial plexus from its origin to the terminal branching of its cords. The cervicothoracic parts of the sympathetic trunk can be exposed by displacing the suprapleural membrane from the first rib. On the left side the terminal thoracic duct is exposed as it ascends along the left side of the esophagus and arches over the pleura between the carotid sheath in front and the subclavian artery behind (see Fig. 133).

Transthoracic control of a large vessel may sometimes be obviated by the retrograde insertion of an intravascular balloon catheter.

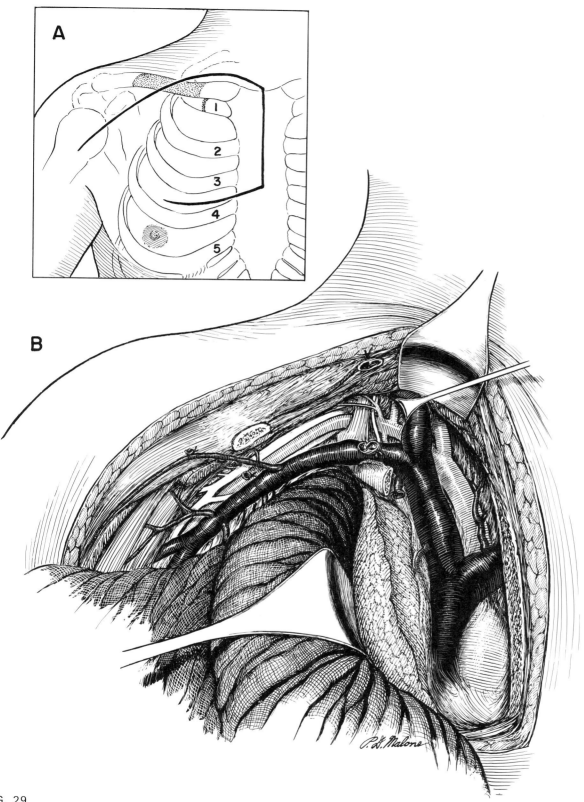

FIG. 29
Cervicothoracic-axillary exposure.

REFERENCES

Amato, J. J., Vanecko, R. M., Yao, S. T., and Weinberg, M., Jr.: Emergency approach to the subclavian and innominate vessels. Ann. Thorac. Surg. 8:537–541, 1969.

Blalock, A.: Surgical procedures employed and anatomical variations encountered in the treatment of congenital pulmonic stenosis. Surg. Gynec. Obstet. 87:385–409, 1948.

Henry, A. K.: Extensile Exposure, 2nd ed. Edinburgh, Livingstone, 1957.

Kerr, H. H., and Warfield, J. O., Jr.: Intrathoracic dermoids. With the report of a case of total extirpation at one sitting by a new method of thoracotomy. Ann. Surg. 88:607–629, 1928.

Killian, H.: Aneurysmen des brachiocephalen Stromgebietes und weitere Erfahrungen mit der Mediastinotomia sternoclavicularis. Langenbecks Arch. u. Dtsch. Z. Chir. 269:200–214, 1951.

Mansberger, A. R., Jr., and Linberg, E. J.: First rib resection for distal exposure of subclavian vessels. Surg. Gynec. Obstet. 120:578–579, 1965.

Sencert, L.: Les blessures des gros troncs vasculaires de la base du cou et leur traitement chirurgical. J. Chir. 15:101–135, 1918.

Webb, W. R., and Burford, T. H.: Gangrene of the arm following use of the subclavian artery in a pulmonosystemic (Blalock) anastomosis. J. Thor. Surg. 23:199–204, 1952.

Yao, J. K. Y., and Mustard, W. T.: An extrapleural approach to the heart with particular reference to pulmonary artery banding and innominate artery suspension. J. Cardiovasc. Surg. 10:273, 1969.

CONGENITAL AbNORMALITIES of THE GREAT VESSELS

DERIVATION OF ANOMALIES OF THE AORTA AND OF VASCULAR RINGS

The system of aortic arches of the mammalian embryo, which forms the basis for development of the thoracic aorta and its branches, are shown in the so-called Rathke diagram in Figure 30. J. E. Edwards (1953) created his own representation, which presents more clearly the gross anatomy of man, and forms the basis for ready classification of anomalies encountered. Figure 31 I shows his primitive hypothetical stage in which there exists a complete aortic vascular ring about the trachea and esophagus. The ascending aorta is connected to the descending aorta by segments of the ring identifiable as right and left aortic arches (rather than the earlier multiple-numbered arches).

In an intermediate hypothetical stage (Figure 31 II) a double arch is still present. Four basic derivations are possible, according to deviation of the descending aorta to the right or left, and disappearance of one or the other ductus.

The development of a final 'normal' pattern is shown in Figure 31 III-a. The descending aorta has deviated to the left, and the left ductus remains. The right aortic arch has dropped out. The demarcation of this disappearance is indi-

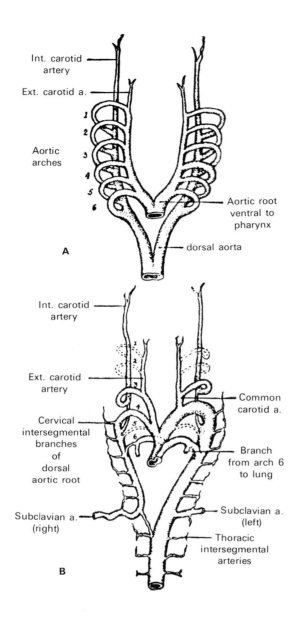

Int. carotid artery

Ext. carotid a.

Aortic arches

1
2
3
4
5
6

Aortic root ventral to pharynx

dorsal aorta

A

Int. carotid artery

Ext. carotid artery

Common carotid a.

Cervical intersegmental branches of dorsal aortic root

Branch from arch 6 to lung

Subclavian a. (right)

Subclavian a. (left)

Thoracic intersegmental arteries

B

FIG. 30
Aortic arches of mammalian embryo. A. Ground plan. B. Early modification. (From Patten, 1968.)

cated by the line across the aortic ring shown in Figure 31 III-b. Figure 31 IV shows the production of a retro-esophageal right subclavian artery by the anomalous line of interruption distal to the origin of the subclavian artery. The persistent left posterior part of the aortic ring now constitutes the origin of the right subclavian artery. Figure 38 shows this vessel segment, reduced in caliber, persisting as an arteria aberrans, while the subclavian takes its usual origin. The association of non-recurrence of the inferior laryngeal nerve with a retro-esophageal subclavian artery is discussed in Chapter 8. Anomalies of other arteries (pp. 82–83), and

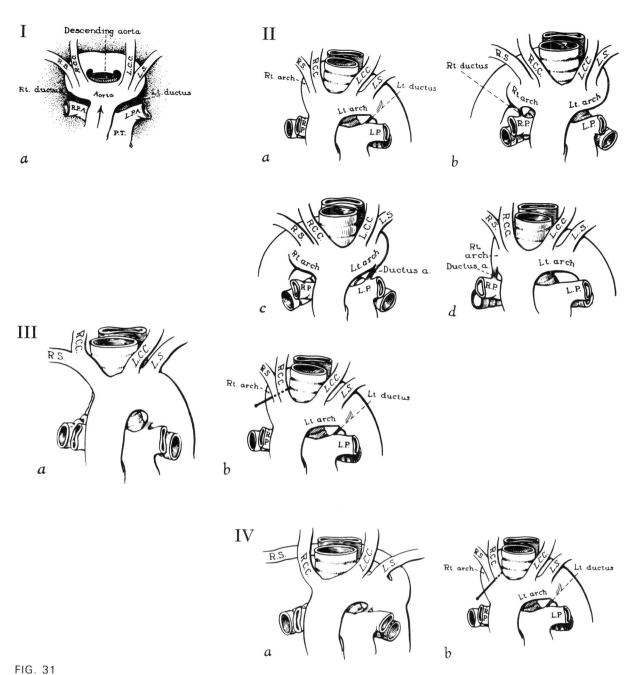

FIG. 31

Derivation of aorta and vascular rings.   I. Hypothetical primitive aortic plan.   II. Four derived double-arch systems. III. (a) Usual adult pattern.   (b) Double arch system (as in IIa), normally interrupted at line shown. When this system persists as a vascular ring, the ring may be surgically divided at the same line.   IV. (a) Retro-esophageal right subclavian artery.   (b) The production of this anomaly by developmental interruption of the basic arch system between the right common carotid and right subclavian arteries. (From Edwards, 1953.)

of the thoracic duct (p. 231), may be associated. It should be noted that vascular rings may be ligamentous in whole or in part.

VASCULAR RINGS

Operations on anomalies of the aortic arch system, expressed as vascular rings, are done to relieve compression of the trachea, esophagus, or, rarely, as in right aortic arch, an upper lobe bronchus. Relief in these instances is obtained in one of three ways: (1) by division of the constricting vessel, (2) by relaxation of the ring by division of a taut ductus arteriosus (or ligament), or (3) by changing the course of a constricting vessel by fixing it to a neighboring structure. An obstructing retro-esophageal subclavian artery is divided, preferably at its origin.

The smaller of two aortic arches, usually the left or anterior, may be divided. An anterior vessel, constrictive because of an unusual angle of course, as a brachiocephalic trunk arising too far to the left, or a left common carotid artery arising from a point to the right of the midline, may be lifted off the trachea by tacking it to the back of the sternum (Fig. 32).

When, in the presence of a single arch, the pulmonary artery compresses the trachea, division of the ductus may allow the pulmonary artery to fall away from the trachea. Edwards *et al.* (1948) state that the structure to be divided either is the ductus or lies on the same side as the ductus. For this reason it is advised that the thoracotomy should be

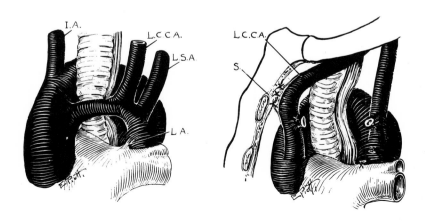

FIG. 32
Division of vascular ring and suspension of the left common carotid artery. (From Gross, 1947.)

done on that side. The ductus is usually present on the side of the descending aorta, a fact often determined by x-ray examination.

Gross (1953) advises a left anterolateral incision through the third intercostal space regardless of the type of vascular ring to be treated. Anterior mediastinal dissection is necessary in double aortic arch, right arch with left ductus, anomalous brachiocephalic trunk, and anomalous left common carotid artery. He advises removal of much of the thymus, avoiding injury to the brachiocephalic veins or the right pleura. For aberrant subclavian artery only the posterior mediastinum need be opened, dissecting behind the aortic arch and the vagus nerves, sparing the recurrent left laryngeal nerve.

Some anomalies require extensive posterior as well as anterior mediastinal dissection, even to the right of the spine. The thoracic duct must be identified (see Fig. 17) and spared. Suspension of the brachiocephalic trunk has been done extrapleurally through the left second intercostal space anteriorly (Yao and Mustard, 1969).

Compression of the trachea by abnormal pulmonary arteries in association with congenital heart disease is recorded by Park *et al.* (1971).

PATENT DUCTUS ARTERIOSUS

Gross (1953) advises an anterolateral approach through the third intercostal space, cutting the intercostal muscles all the way to the angles of the ribs, and reserving a posterior approach for the rare patient with a huge ductus in whom it may be necessary to apply a circumaortic clamp to isolate the ductus. King and Mandelbaum (1962) have used an extrapleural approach to the ductus through the fourth intercostal space posterolaterally.

The ductus passes from the left side of the bifurcation of the pulmonary trunk to the concavity of the junction of the arch and descending aorta (Fig. 33). The vagus nerve is the guide to the lower border of the ductus. It can be seen through the pleura, crossing the aorta and lateral part of the ductus, here to run behind the pulmonary root. The recurrent laryngeal nerve is given off from the vagus at the

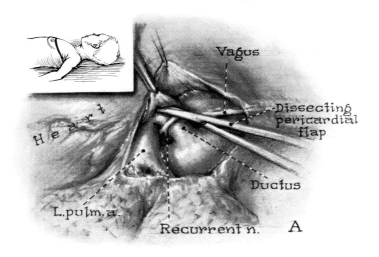

FIG. 33
Exposure of patent ductus arteriosus.
(*From Bahnson, in Gibbon* et al.,
1969.)

inferior edge of the ductus to wind medially round it. Here the nerve gives off inferior cardiac branches as it begins to ascend on the posterior edge of the trachea.

COARCTATION OF THE AORTA

Coarctation usually involves the aorta just beyond the origin of the left subclavian artery, either proximal or distal to the ductus. Special anatomical interest in coarctation relates to the enlargement of certain vessels as collaterals (Edwards, 1948) (Fig. 34), and the consequences of temporary or permanent interference with the blood supply of the spinal cord (pp. 73 *et seq.*).

Gross (1953) used a posterolateral T-shaped exposure, obtained by opening the fourth intercostal space in its entire length, with posterior division of two ribs and intercostal bundles above and two or three ribs and intercostal bundles below (Fig. 35). The 'ascending branch' of the transverse cervical artery lies beneath the trapezius, and the 'descending branch' of the same vessel lies beneath the rhomboids (see Fig. 7). The latissimus dorsi and intercostal muscles will be unusually vascular. Anteriorly (Fig. 35) the incision runs up to the much enlarged internal thoracic (internal mammary) artery, which should be spared. Some use an anterolateral approach (Fig. 36).

The aorta, the left subclavian artery, and the ductus are mobilized, the left vagus and recurrent laryngeal nerves being retracted. Injury to the thoracic duct is avoided by dissecting close to the aorta (see Fig. 18). Branches arising from the anterior surface of the aorta course to the viscera of the posterior mediastinum, but their exact destination cannot be known from the limited dissection at operation. They include left, and occasionally right, bronchial and esophageal arteries. No certain deleterious effects follow the operative division of these branches of the aorta. Some intercostal arteries may require temporary occlusion. Their division should be avoided because of possible damage to the spinal cord. The blood supply of the thoracic viscera and the cord is considered in detail in Chapter 7.

Schuster and Gross (1962) gave the name 'artery of Abbott' to an anomalous artery arising from the back of the aorta, immediately above the coarctation (Fig. 37), originally described by Hamilton and Abbott in 1928. It courses medially beneath the aortic arch or the carotid artery. This artery may be close to 1 cm in diameter and aneurysmal; its dissection can be hazardous.

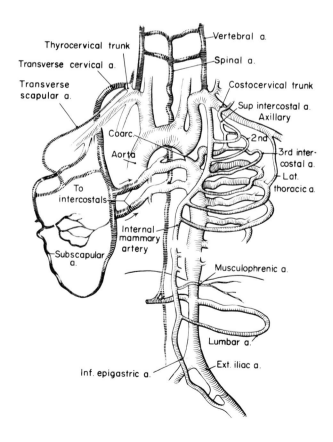

FIG. 34
Collateral circulation in coarctation of the aorta. Two main pathways are apparent: (1) The parascapular arteries are the major affluent vessels to the intercostal arteries and thence to the abdominal viscera. Characteristically, the aorta narrows again below the renal arteries. (2) The internal thoracic artery appears to be the major source of blood to the lower limb, since the external iliac artery widens below its junction with the inferior epigastric artery. (Edwards, 1971.)

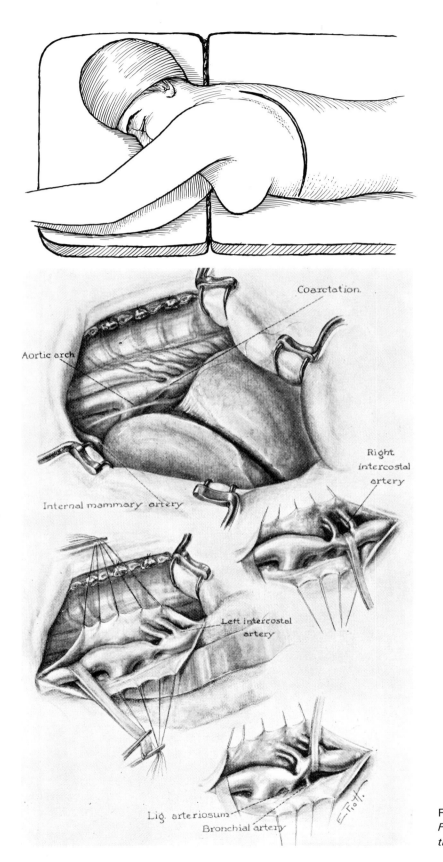

Coarctation.

Aortic arch

Right intercostal artery

Internal mammary artery

Left intercostal artery

Lig. arteriosum

Bronchial artery

E. Toff.

FIG. 35
Posterolateral exposure for coarctation of the aorta. (From Gross, 1953.)

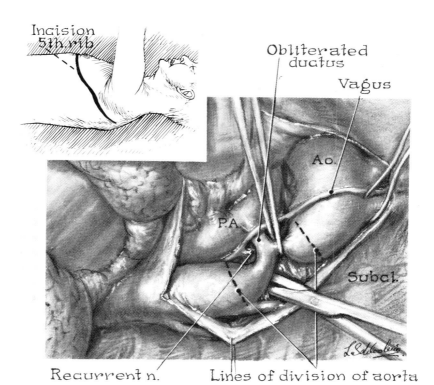

FIG. 36
Anterolateral exposure for coarctation of the aorta. Subcl. refers to the subclavian artery encircled by the tape. (From Bahnson, in Gibbon et al., 1969.)

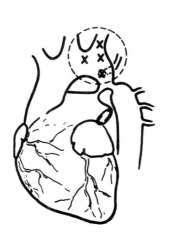

FIG. 37
Sites of origin of 'Abbott's artery.' (From Schuster and Gross, 1962.) Xs indicate sites on posterior wall of aorta where Schuster and Gross observed origin of this anomalous vessel.

REFERENCES

Bahnson, H. T.: The Aortic Arch and the Thoracic Aorta. Chapter 23 *in* Surgery of the Chest, Gibbon, J. H., Jr., Sabiston, D. C., Jr., and Spencer, F. C., Eds., 2nd ed. Philadelphia, W. B. Saunders, 1969.

Edwards, J. E.: Anomalies of the derivatives of the aortic arch system. Med. Clin. N. Amer. 32:925–949, 1948.

Edwards, J. E.: Malformations of the aortic arch system manifested as "vascular rings." Lab. Invest. 2:56–75, 1953.

Edwards, J. E.: Personal communication, 1971.

Edwards, J. E., Clagett, O. T., Drake, R. L., and Christensen, N. A.: The collateral circulation in coarctation of the aorta. Proc. Staff Meet. Mayo. Clin. 23:333–339, 1948.

Gross, R. E.: Surgical Treatment for Abnormalities of the Heart and Great Vessels. Springfield, Charles C Thomas, 1947.

Gross, R. E.: The Surgery of Infancy and Childhood. Its Principles and Techniques. Philadelphia, W. B. Saunders, 1953.

Hamilton, W. F., and Abbott, M. E.: Coarctation of the aorta of the adult type. I. Complete obliteration of the descending arch at insertion of the ductus in a boy of fourteen; bicuspid aortic valve; impending rupture of the aorta, cerebral death. Amer. Heart J. 3:381–392, 1928.

King, H., and Mandelbaum, I.: Extrapleural approach for patent ductus arteriosus. Surgery 51:277–279, 1962.

Park, C. D., Waldhausen, J. A., Friedman, S., Aberdeen, E., and Johnson, J.: Tracheal compression by the great arteries in the mediastinum. Reports of 39 cases. Arch. Surg. 103:626–632, 1971.

Patten, B. M.: Human Embryology, 3rd ed. New York, McGraw-Hill, 1968.

Schuster, S. R., and Gross, R. E.: Surgery for coarctation of the aorta. A review of 500 cases. J. Thorac. Cardiovasc. Surg. 43:54–70, 1962.

Yao, J. K. Y., and Mustard, W. T.: An extrapleural approach to the heart with particular reference to pulmonary artery banding and innominate artery suspension. J. Cardiovasc. Surg. 10:273, 1969.

VASCULAR SUPPLY OF THE THORACIC VISCERA, EXCLUSIVE OF THE CORONARY AND PULMONARY VESSELS

This Chapter will consider the interrelationship of arteries and veins of the mediastinal viscera, spinal cord, large nerves, and the bronchial territory.

MAIN ARTERIAL SOURCES

The subclavian artery and the descending thoracic aorta are the major sources of oxygenated blood to the thoracic viscera, with assistance from the esophageal branches of the left gastric and inferior phrenic arteries. Anomalously some branches may also come from the brachiocephalic trunk. The bronchial and intercostal arteries constitute important inter-mediaries.

The two largest visceral branches of the subclavian artery are the vertebral and the inferior thyroid artery (see Fig. 1). The vertebral arteries share with the internal carotid arteries the supply of the brain and, through the anterior spinal arteries and irregular spinal branches, constitute the sole supply to the cervical cord. Variations in origin, size, and course of the vertebral arteries are considered in Chapter 4 and Figures 23, 24. In addition to supplying, with the superior thyroid arteries, the larynx and the thyroid and parathyroid glands, the inferior thyroid arteries contribute almost the entire supply to the lower pharynx, trachea, cervical esophagus, and, inconstantly, the thymus. The internal thoracic arteries give the most constant branches to the thymus (see Fig. 55). The pericardiacophrenic artery and smaller branches supply the mediastinal pleura and pericardium, with collateral branches to the coronary tree. Perforating branches of the anterior intercostal arteries supply the breast (see Fig. 39). The superior intercostal branch of the costocervical trunk gives off the first two posterior intercostal arteries sharing in the visceral distribution of the aortic intercostal arteries.

The descending thoracic aorta provides branches to the trachea, bronchi, esophagus, vagal and sympathetic plexuses, the spinal cord, and breast. These branches are partly direct and partly via the posterior intercostal and bronchial branches of the aorta.

THE INTERCOSTAL ARTERIES

For each intercostal space there exists one posterior intercostal artery. The superior intercostal artery from the costocervical trunk usually supplies the first two intercostal spaces. The descending aorta gives off nine intercostal vessels: the first is usually the third intercostal artery. The costocervical trunk and the proximal part of the descending aorta may be connected by a slender arteria aberrans (Fig. 38), the remnant of the right dorsal aorta, and a replica of the anomalous retro-esophageal subclavian artery (see Fig. 49). The posterior intercostal arteries give posterior branches directed toward the intervertebral foramina, particularly important as the source of the arteries to the spinal cord (p. 73). The intercostal artery then joins the intercostal nerve to run under cover of the groove of the rib, above each intercostal space. Anteriorly, the intercostal artery and its collateral branch (coursing in the lower part of the intercostal space) anastomose with the anterior intercostal arteries.

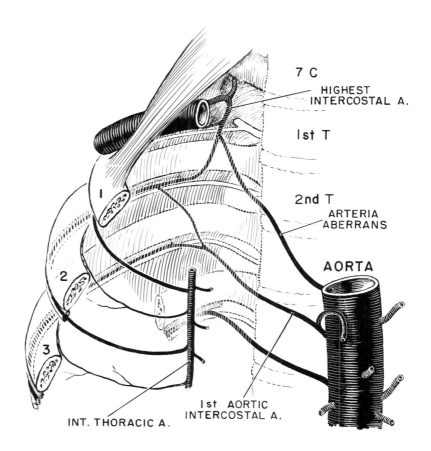

FIG. 38
Plan of the intercostal arteries. (After Walsham in Anson, 1966.)

These anterior intercostal arteries stem from the internal thoracic artery and its musculophrenic branch. They are small and irregular in number, one or two being given off in each space (Fig. 38). Visceral branches of the intercostal arteries (Fig. 39) include the arteries to the thoracic spinal cord (through irregularly placed anterior and posterior radicular branches of the primary posterior branches), the right and occasionally a left bronchial branch from right intercostal arteries, usually the first aortic (third posterior) intercostal; esophageal, tracheal, and 'mediastinal' branches to pleura, lymph nodes, and nerves; and perforating lateral and medial branches to the breast.

THE BRONCHIAL ARTERIES

Most commonly the right lung is supplied by a single bronchial artery arising from the first right aortic intercostal artery (Fig. 40). The right bronchial artery may occasionally

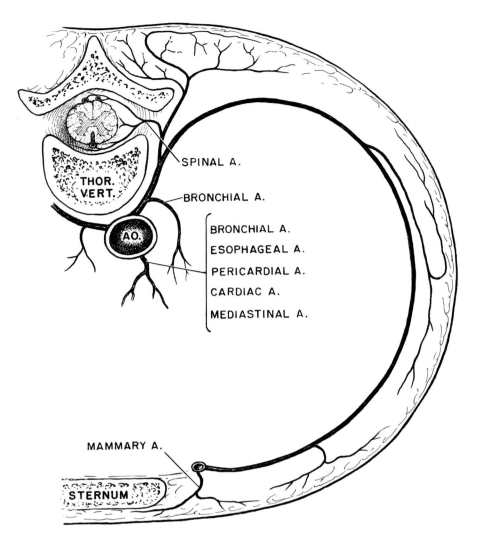

SPINAL A.

THOR.
VERT.

BRONCHIAL A.

AO.

BRONCHIAL A.
ESOPHAGEAL A.
PERICARDIAL A.
CARDIAC A.
MEDIASTINAL A.

MAMMARY A.

STERNUM

FIG. 39
*Visceral branches of an intercostal
artery.*

arise from the aorta, in common with a left superior bronchial
artery, or more rarely from the aorta independently. There
are usually two left bronchial arteries arising from the beginning of the descending aorta, the superior to the upper lobe
and the inferior to the lower lobe (Fig. 41). Cauldwell *et al.*
(1948) found that a left bronchial artery may arise from a
right intercostal artery but no bronchial artery was found
originating from any left intercostal artery except in one case
of situs inversus. At least one bronchial artery, a right or
a left, came directly from the aorta in every specimen ex-
amined.

Anomalously, bronchial arteries may arise from the subclavian artery or any of its branches, especially the internal
thoracic or the superior intercostal branch of the costocervical

trunk. In a case reported by O'Rahilly *et al.* (1950) a bronchial artery arising from the latter vessel ran anterior to the trachea and was the sole bronchial supply to both lungs. Menke (1936) illustrated a huge right bronchial artery arising from the right subclavian artery, descending on the anterior aspect of the trachea and supplemented by a smaller right

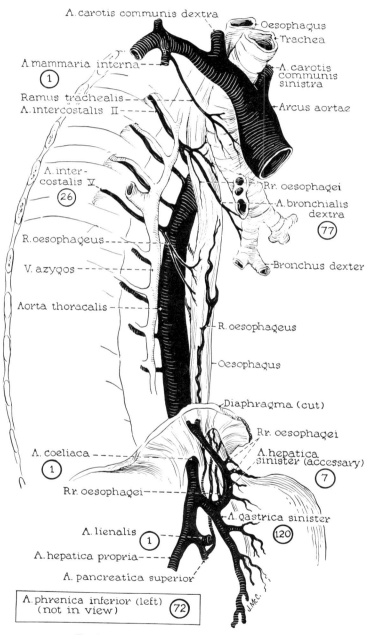

Esophageal and bronchial arteries; diagrammatic.

The encircled numbers near the labelled vessel record the frequency of origin of esophageal rami from the particular vessel in 125 specimens.

FIG. 40
Bronchial and esophageal arteries, right view. (From Swigart et al., *1950.)*

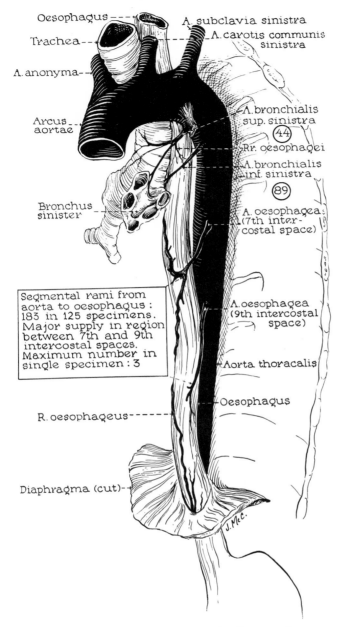

Oesophagus

Trachea

A. anonyma

Arcus
aortae

Bronchus
sinister

A. subclavia sinistra

A. carotis communis
sinistra

A. bronchialis
sup. sinistra

44

Rr. oesophagei

A. bronchialis
inf. sinistra

89

A. oesophagea
(7th inter-
costal space)

A. oesophagea
(9th intercostal
space)

Aorta thoracalis

Oesophagus

Segmental rami from
aorta to oesophagus:
183 in 125 specimens.
Major supply in region
between 7th and 9th
intercostal spaces.
Maximum number in
single specimen: 3

R. oesophageus

Diaphragma (cut)

J. McC.

Thoracic sources of esophageal arteries; diagrammatic.

The encircled numbers represent the frequency with which esophageal rami arose from the particular bronchial
artery in 125 dissections. Ascending branches of esophageal arteries from abdominal level and descending branches
of the segmental esophageal arteries of thoracic level are also shown.

FIG. 41
*Bronchial and esophageal arteries,
left view. (From Swigart et al.,
1950.)*

bronchial artery from an intercostal (Fig. 42). The bronchial
arteries generally course on the posterior aspect of their
respective bronchi. However, the right bronchial artery, especially when arising from an unusual source, may travel
anterior to the trachea or the esophagus (8.7 per cent as
reported by Cauldwell *et al.* 1948). Nathan *et al.* (1970)

suggest that the right bronchial artery of usual origin may be located surgically by retracting the arch of the azygos vein, whose course it parallels.

The bronchial arteries have a wide distribution. Not only do they supply the hilum of the lung, as well as the lung parenchyma, but they quite routinely give branches to all the posterior mediastinal structures. The bronchial arteries thus constitute the major supply to the thoracic trachea and the upper part of the thoracic esophagus. They also give contributions to the pericardium, atria (thus communicating with the coronary arteries [p. 146]), and the vagus and sympathetic plexuses. Conversely, Cauldwell *et al.* (1948) cite accessory bronchial vessels which arise from esophageal arteries and course through the pulmonary ligaments. Major anastomoses may connect the main bronchial arteries.

The bronchial arteries are much enlarged in conditions in which pulmonary artery flow is restricted, as in pulmonic

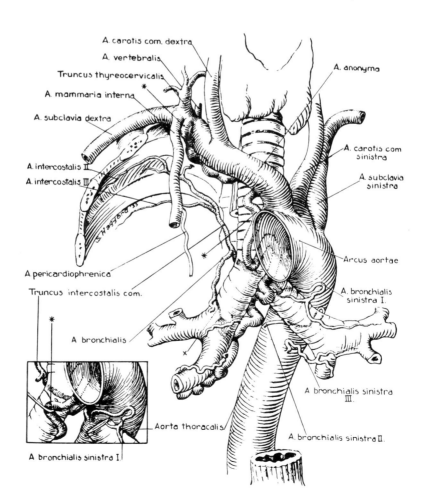

FIG. 42
Anomalous right bronchial artery. The anomalous bronchial artery (*) arises from the right subclavian artery. A second right and one left bronchial artery course from the truncus intercostalis com. of aortic origin (insert). The two right bronchial arteries communicate at X. Two left bronchial arteries arise from the aorta. (From Menke, 1936.)

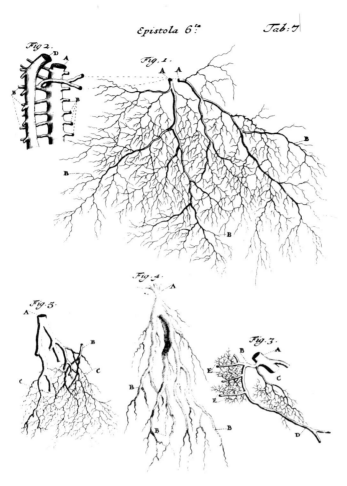

Epistola 6.ª   *Tab: 7*

Fig. 2.   *Fig. 1.*   *Fig. 5.*   *Fig. 4.*   *Fig. 3.*

FIG. 43

Bronchial arteries and bronchial–pulmonary artery communications. Delineation by wax injection into the pulmonary artery in human infants. 'Fig 1.' Arborization of the bronchial arteries. 'Fig 2.' Origin of the (right?) bronchial artery from a right aortic intercostal. A is the aorta, D, the azygos vein. 'Fig. 3.' Origin of the (right?) bronchial artery, D, from the superior intercostal artery, B, stemming from the subclavian, A. C is an 'esophageal artery, arising from the intercostal, and heretofore neglected by anatomists,' E, pleural branches. 'Fig 4.' 'Coagulated blood serum, commonly called a polyp, expectorated from the wind-pipe.' This concerned a separate issue discussed in the same paper. 'Fig. 5.' A. A branch of the pulmonary artery. B. A branch of the bronchial artery, filled through inosculations, C, between the two. (From Ruysch, 1696.)

stenosis. In such conditions oxygenation is carried out via the bronchial artery–pulmonary artery anastomoses, already known to Ruysch in 1696 (Fig. 43). They may be greatly enlarged in inflammatory or neoplastic disease of the lungs. Extensive occlusion of the bronchial arterial tree in the dog (Ellis *et al.*, 1951) results in bronchopulmonary ulceration and death. Simple ligation, as in pneumonectomy, has given no observable effect.

ARTERIES TO ESOPHAGUS AND TRACHEA

For purposes of description the esophagus may be divided into four parts: the cervical; the upper thoracic, or 'pars bifurcalis'; the lower thoracic; and the abdominal. Only the lower thoracic esophagus receives arteries for that organ alone; the other segments share their arteries with adjacent structures (Demel, 1924; Shapiro and Robillard, 1950; Swigart et al., 1950).

The abdominal segment is supplied by a number of branches from the left gastric artery, often supplemented by branches from the left inferior phrenic artery, or from the left hepatic when that vessel takes origin from the left gastric. Infrequently a major esophageal vessel may arise from the left inferior phrenic artery.

The 'esophageal arteries' for the lower thoracic segment are likely to be few in number but larger than in other regions (see Figs. 40 and 41). There are usually two unpaired esophageal arteries arising from the aorta (range 0 to 3, according to Swigart et al. 1950). Those of the left side tend to be the larger. In 20 per cent Swigart et al. found them augmented by one or more esophageal arteries from a right intercostal artery, often the fifth. Esophageal branches from left intercostal arteries were rare. The arteries to the lower thoracic segment, more than elsewhere, tend to bifurcate on the organ, to communicate with the arteries of the segments above and below.

The upper thoracic segment lies to the right of and above the arch of the aorta. It is often called the 'pars bifurcalis' because of its relationship to the thoracic trachea and the bronchi, whose arteries it shares. The major arterial supply is from the bronchial arteries of both sides. Rarely there exist branches from the aorta or from the subclavian artery or its branches.

The cervical esophagus is supplied by three tracheo-esophageal branches of the inferior thyroid artery (Swigart et al., 1950; Miura and Grillo, 1966), of which the inferior is usually the largest, giving a branch which descends along the recurrent laryngeal nerve to anastomose with the bronchial arteries (see Fig. 110). Uncommonly the subclavian artery or its other branches and, rarely, the common carotid or thyroidea ima artery are the source of cervical tracheo-esophageal arteries. At the upper end of the esophagus the vessels anastomose with branches of the superior thyroid and ascending pharyngeal arteries. Arteries of the right side of this segment are said to be the larger.

It is generally recognized that the communications are relatively inadequate at both ends of the cervical esophagus, and at the junction of the lower thoracic and the abdominal segment. The upper end remaining after high thoracic resection is likely to be ischemic unless it is resected high enough to derive good supply from the cervical tracheo-esophageal branches. Shapiro and Robillard (1950) emphasize that where the esophagus shares vessels with those of adjacent organs excessive mobilization is apt to devascularize it. This is especially important for the upper thoracic segment, where mobilization is often bluntly done under the arch of the aorta and where one or two bronchial arteries may be torn.

VISCERAL VEINS

The venous drainage of the thoracic viscera is again remarkable for the interconnection of vessels from the various organs and for the connection between four separate systems: the azygos, vertebral, pulmonary, and portal. The paired azygos and hemiazygos veins are the largest receiving trunks, aided by the brachiocephalic and by the inferior thyroid and other subclavian tributaries. The azygos and vertebral veins communicate via spinal tributaries of the intercostal veins.

The major esophageal drainage is into the azygos and hemiazygos veins, with a small vein accompanying each vagus nerve (Fig. 44). In the superior mediastinum, as in the neck, the esophageal veins end in the inferior thyroid and other vessels and are well connected with the tracheal veins. At their inferior end the esophageal veins connect with the coronary vein. Many communications exist along the esophagus between its veins and other tributaries of the azygos system.

The bronchial veins terminate in the azygos vessels, but within the lung they are extensively connected with the pulmonary venous radicles. In those rare instances of survival after apparent complete embolic obstruction of the pulmonary arteries, systemic venous blood is shunted to the pulmonary veins and the left heart via the bronchial veins, while oxygenation is carried out through the bronchial arteries via their communications with the pulmonary arteries.

The communications between the left gastric and esophageal veins explain the presence of esophageal varices in portal obstruction and the rationale for esophagogastric re-

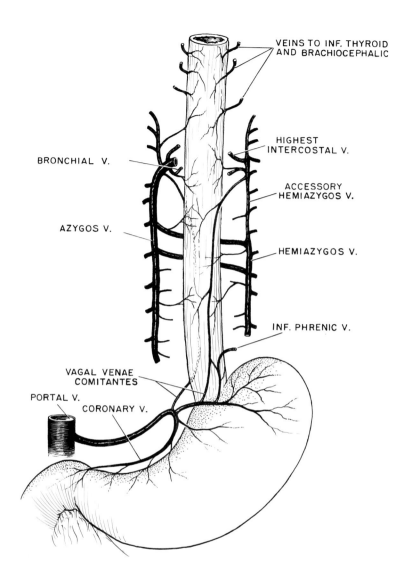

Labels in figure:
VEINS TO INF. THYROID AND BRACHIOCEPHALIC
HIGHEST INTERCOSTAL V.
ACCESSORY HEMIAZYGOS V.
HEMIAZYGOS V.
INF. PHRENIC V.
BRONCHIAL V.
AZYGOS V.
VAGAL VENAE COMITANTES
PORTAL V.
CORONARY V.

FIG. 44
Venous drainage of the esophagus.
(After Butler, 1951, and Hollinshead, 1956.)

section or venous ligature in this territory (Linton and Warren, 1953). Other observations also indicate the possibility of spontaneous portapulmonary venous shunting via the intermediary of posterior mediastinal and bronchial veins (Blackburn, 1956).

THE VASCULAR SUPPLY OF THE SPINAL CORD

The spinal cord is supplied by a limited number of arteries and veins, and communications between its various levels may be quite inadequate. The single anterior spinal artery is usually bold in the cervical and even larger in the lumbar part of the cord, but is tenuous in the thoracic region where it may consist of small anastomoses between the several radicular branches of the intercostal arteries. The posterior spinal arteries are usually a paired set of intersegmental communications. The arteries of the cord are contributed to quite constantly by the intracranial and the upper one or two cervical levels of the vertebral arteries, but the widest part of the anterior spinal artery, that at the lumbar segments, receives the 'arteria radicularis magna' from the segmental artery of one side or the other. The source of the arteria radicularis magna is most frequently a second lumbar artery, but there is a range of origin from the eighth thoracic to the fourth lumbar (Suh and Alexander, 1939).

There are *potential* contributions of anterior and posterior radicular branches at all vertebral levels, stemming from the vertebral arteries in the neck, the superior intercostal branch of the costovertebral trunk for the upper two intercostal segments, and the aortic intercostal and lumbar arteries for the remainder. The *actual* supply is only by six to eight anterior radicular and five to eight posterior radicular arteries (Suh and Alexander, 1939) (Fig. 45).

The veins join a larger posterior and a smaller anterior trunk with exits from the vertebral column via 5 to 10 posterior and 6 to 11 anterior radicular veins (Fig. 45). Again the largest vein ('vena radicularis magna') is in the lumbar or lower thoracic region, more often on the left side (Suh and Alexander, 1939).

The thoracic part of the cord is most frequently damaged by arterial or venous interruption: first because the vessels that supply it are the smallest, and second because it is farthest away from the larger cervical and lumbar sources of supply. Such an area is one which Edwards (1958) has called a 'junctional zone' (the 'border zone' of neurologists).

Paraplegia after aortic surgery has most often occurred when the procedure has been performed on the thoracic aorta. To some degree it is the consequence of temporary occlusion of the aorta or of a segmental artery (Adams and van Geertruyden, 1956), but division of an intercostal or lumbar vessel which happens to give off a preponderant artery to the cord often appears responsible. Paraplegia has occurred after operations for coarctation or aneurysm of the thoracic aorta (Adams and van Geertruyden, 1956), lumbo-

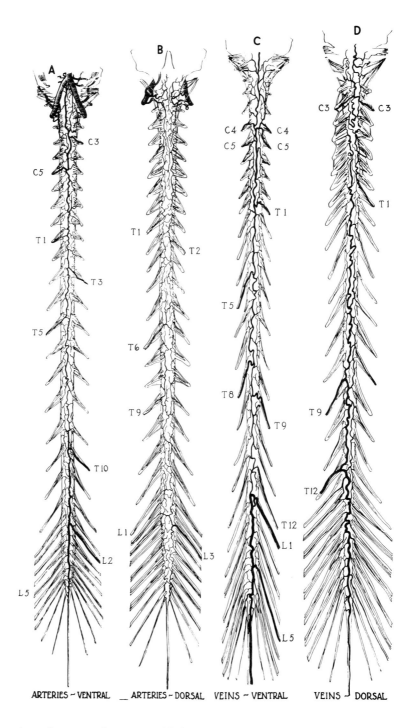

ARTERIES ~ VENTRAL __ ARTERIES ~ DORSAL VEINS ~ VENTRAL VEINS _| DORSAL

FIG. 45
Vessels of the human spinal cord, drawn to scale; based on data from 26 cases. (From Suh and Alexander, 1939.)

dorsal sympathectomy (Adams and van Geertruyden, 1956; Hughes and Macintyre, 1963), and after resection of abdominal aortic aneurysm (Skillman *et al.*, 1969). It has also followed bronchial arteriography, presumably because of filling of a significant intercostal artery by the vasographic medium. We have seen one case in which paraplegia followed aortography and excessive filling of a left eleventh intercostal artery. Suh and Alexander (1939) give examples of cord injury from venous occlusion, but the results of occlusion of individual veins are less well documented than those of occlusion of the arteries.

References

Adams, H. D., and van Geertruyden, H. H.: Neurologic complications of aortic surgery. Trans. Amer. Surg. Assn. 74:281–317, 1956.

Blackburn, C. R. B.: Acquired portal-pulmonary venous anastomosis complicating partial oesophago-gastrectomy in a patient with portal hypertension. Thorax 11:30–35, 1956.

Butler, H.: The veins of the oesophagus. Thorax 6:276–296, 1951.

Cauldwell, E. W., Siekert, R. G., Lininger, R. E., and Anson, B. J.: The bronchial arteries. An anatomic study of 150 human cadavers. Surg. Gynec. Obstet. 86:395–412, 1948.

Demel, R.: Die Gefässversorgung der Speiseröhre. Ein Beitrag zur Oesophaguschirurgie. Arch. Klin. Chir. 128:453–504, 1924.

Edwards, E. A.: The anatomy of collateral circulation. Surg. Gynec. Obstet. 107:183–194, 1958.

Ellis, F. H., Jr., Grindlay, J. H., and Edwards, J. E.: The bronchial arteries. I. Experimental occlusion. Surgery 30:810–826, 1951.

Hollinshead, W. H.: Anatomy for Surgeons. Vol. 2, The Thorax, Abdomen, and Pelvis, New York, Paul B. Hoeber, Inc., 1956.

Hughes, J. T., and Macintyre, A. G.: Spinal cord infarction occurring during thoraco-lumbar sympathectomy. J. Neurol. Neurosurg. Psychiat. 26:418–421, 1963.

Linton, R. R., and Warren, R.: The emergency treatment of massive bleeding from esophageal varices by transesophageal suture of these vessels at the time of acute hemorrhage. Surgery 33:243–255, 1953.

Menke, J. F.: An anomalous a. bronchialis dextra from the a. subclavia dextra, secondarily connected to the aorta thoracalis. Anat. Rec. 65:55–58, 1936.

Miura, T., and Grillo, H. C.: The contribution of the inferior thyroid artery to the blood supply of the human trachea. Surg. Gynec. Obstet. 123:99–102, 1966.

Mohr, P. D.: The blood supply of the vagus nerve. Acta Anat. 73:19–26, 1969.

Nathan, H., Orda, R., and Barkay, M.: The right bronchial artery. Anatomical considerations and surgical approach. Thorax 25:328–333, 1970.

O'Rahilly, R., Debson, H., and King, T. S.: Subclavian origin of bronchial arteries. Anat. Rec. 108:227–238, 1950.

Ruysch, F.: Epistola Anatomica, Problematica Sexta. Amstelaedami, Joannem Wolters, 1696. *In* Opera Omnia, Amstelaedami, Janssonio-Waesbergios, 1721.

Shapiro, A. L., and Robillard, G. L.: The esophageal arteries. Their configurational anatomy and variations in relation to surgery. Ann. Surg. 131:171–185, 1950.

Skillman, J. J., Zervas, N. T., Weintraub, R. M., and Mayman, C. I.: Paraplegia after resection of aneurysms of the abdominal aorta. New Eng. J. Med. 281:422–425, 1969.

Suh, T. H., and Alexander, L.: Vascular system of the human spinal cord. Arch. Neurol. Psychiat. 41:659–677, 1939.

Swigart, L. L., Siekert, R. G., Hambley, W. C., and Anson, B. J.: The esophageal arteries. An anatomic study of 150 specimens. Surg. Gynec. Obstet. 90:234–243, 1950.

Thoracic Aspects of Thyroid, Parathyroids, and Thymus

INTRATHORACIC GOITER

Some or all of a goiter may be located within the thorax, commonly in the substernal position, rarely in the posterior mediastinum. Lahey and Swinton (1934) emphasized that the taper of the chest, once the substernal part of the thyroid enlarges, tends to force the mass farther downward in the anterior mediastinum. When the bulk of the goiter lies below the thoracic inlet, the goiter may truly be called intrathoracic. This part of the mass, derived from the lower parts of the thyroid, depends from the inferior thyroid artery, and is usually deliverable from a cervical incision. Sternotomy is required when the thyroid cannot be comfortably delivered from above. Sternotomy may also be necessary for adequate exposure in performing radical thyroidectomy for carcinoma when the gland lies within the thoracic inlet (Fig. 46). It is not done for mediastinal extension of the carcinoma, it being generally understood that the extension is infiltrative and not contained behind a distinct cleavage plane.

The migration of thyroid masses is comparable to that of parathyroid tumors (see Fig. 52). As Sweet (1949) has emphasized, those substernal goiters that arise from the inferior part of the gland descend in front of the trachea,

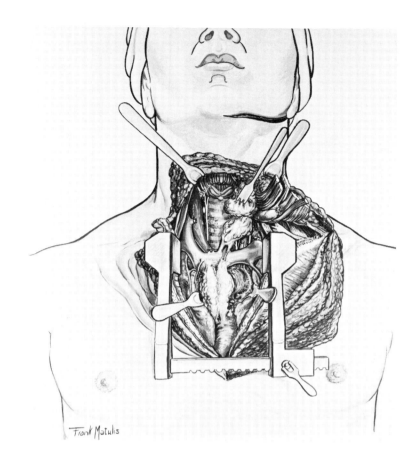

FIG. 46
Cervicothoracic exposure for cancer of the thyroid gland. The collar incision is met by a median sternotomy. The left submandibular incision allows a radical neck dissection to be completed. (From Tamoney, 1970.)

esophagus, and recurrent laryngeal nerve, and lower down are anterior to the great vessels of the superior mediastinum. Only a few thyroid masses originating in this manner descend into the posterior superior mediastinum.

Posterior mediastinal goiters are rare, and their reported relationships are somewhat varied. Falor *et al.* (1955) report that they may have no connection with the cervical thyroid, a condition they characterize as 'primary intrathoracic goiter.' In most reported cases a stalk was found extending downward from the upper lateral part of the cervical gland. Posterior mediastinal goiters are mainly right sided. It is assumed that the aortic arch forces the intrathoracic migration to the right. This is in agreement with the occasional finding of a right intrathoracic goiter connected to the left side of the thyroid gland (Bugden *et al.*, 1959).

Most descriptions of the relationships of posterior intrathoracic goiters emphasize their being wedged against the upper and medial aspect of the arch of the azygos vein, and behind the great vessels of the superior mediastinum, the

4

carotid sheath, and the recurrent laryngeal nerve (Sweet, 1949). The goiter may lie anterior to the trachea, or between the trachea and esophagus.

Exposure of a posterior intrathoracic goiter is almost invariably best accomplished by a right thoracotomy; the azygos vein often requires division. Those goiters with heavy stalks connected to the thyroid gland usually require an additional cervical incision (Sweet, 1949; Adams, 1950; Falor *et al.,* 1955).

Mention must also be made here of intratracheal goiter. As with mediastinal thyroid masses, an intratracheal goiter usually shows a connection with a gland in its normal location (Randolph *et al.,* 1963).

THE THYROIDEA IMA ARTERY

The thyroidea ima artery may be defined as one that arises from a low source other than the subclavian artery proper and ascends to replace or supplement the inferior

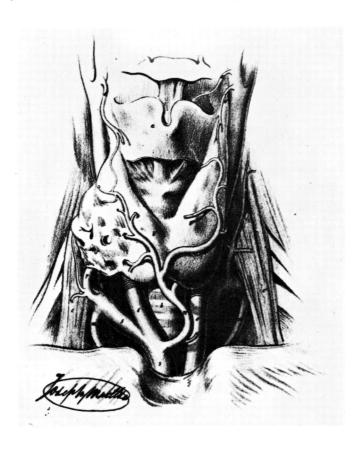

FIG. 47
Thyroidea ima artery arising from the brachiocephalic trunk. (From Quain, 1844.)

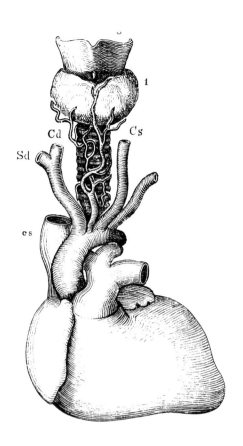

FIG. 48
Thyroidea ima artery arising from the arch of the aorta. (From Henle, 1868.)

thyroid artery. Its incidence is about 10 per cent (Schaeffer, 1953). Most commonly the vessel arises from the brachio-cephalic trunk (Fig. 47). It may arise from the right common carotid or internal thoracic artery, and rarely (about 0.4 per cent) from the arch of the aorta (Fig. 48). When it comes from the aorta it is likely to be a large vessel.

It ascends in front of the trachea, where it is exposed to accidental division in tracheostomy. It generally shows prominent branches on the anterior aspect of the thyroid. Like the inferior thyroid artery, the thyroidea ima artery also supplies branches to the parathyroid glands, the trachea, and the esophagus.

THE RETRO-ESOPHAGEAL SUBCLAVIAN ARTERY AND THE INFERIOR LARYNGEAL NERVE

The usual recurrent course of the inferior laryngeal nerve is based on its embryonic relationship to the aortic arches. The left sixth arch, persisting as the left pulmonary artery and ductus arteriosus, descends in its development, pulling the nerve distally; the nerve then ascends to reach the larynx. On the right, the fifth and sixth arches usually disappear, leaving the nerve in contact with the fourth arch, which gives rise to the usual subclavian artery (see Fig. 30). Thus on the right the nerve passes around the subclavian artery to assume its usual course.

The inferior laryngeal nerve takes a direct rather than a recurrent course in most cases of retro-esophageal origin of the subclavian artery (Fig. 49). It is given off from the vagus nerve at about the level of the superior pole of the thyroid gland and disappears beneath the gland at the middle of its lateral border. There are exceptions. A frequently asso-

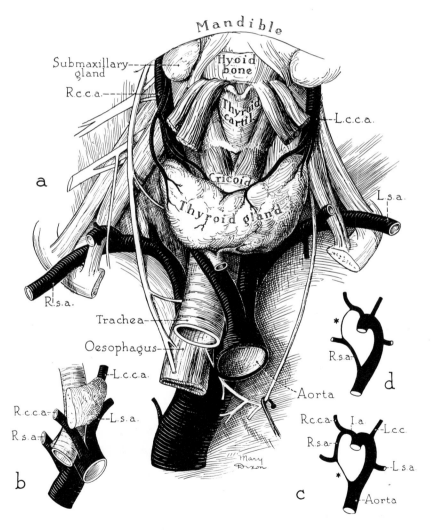

FIG. 49
Descending course of inferior laryngeal nerve with retro-esophageal right subclavian artery. The right inferior laryngeal nerve is apparently indicated in a descending course lateral to the thyroid gland. c. The scheme of origin of the normal subclavian artery from a primitive aortic ring. d. The scheme for the retro-esophageal subclavian artery. (From Anson, 1950.)

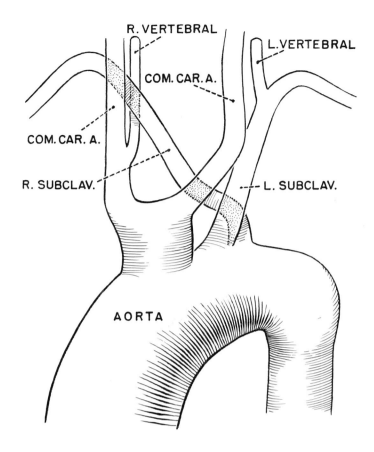

FIG. 50
Retro-esophageal right subclavian artery with anomalous origin of the common carotid and the right vertebral artery, traced from an arch aortogram. The right inferior laryngeal nerve is said to recur about the right vertebral artery in such cases.

ciated arterial anomaly is origin of the vertebral artery of that side from the common carotid artery (Holzapfel, 1899) (Fig. 50). When this is present, the nerve recurs about the vertebral artery. It may also recur about the ductus arteriosus or ligamentum arteriosum (Fig. 51) or about the inferior thyroid artery (Bahnson and Blalock, 1950).

INTRATHORACIC PARATHYROID TUMORS

Parathyroid adenomas may be located within the thorax, those arising from a lower parathyroid gland usually migrating substernally, and those from an upper gland descending into the posterior superior mediastinum (Fig. 52). Only about 10 per cent of adenomas have been found in the thorax, and about twice as many occur in the anterior as in the posterior part of the superior mediastinum.

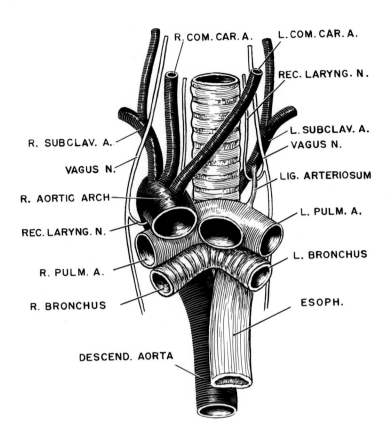

R. COM. CAR. A.
L. COM. CAR. A.
REC. LARYNG. N.
R. SUBCLAV. A.
L. SUBCLAV. A.
VAGUS N.
VAGUS N.
LIG. ARTERIOSUM
R. AORTIC ARCH
L. PULM. A.
REC. LARYNG. N.
R. PULM. A.
L. BRONCHUS
R. BRONCHUS
ESOPH.
DESCEND. AORTA

FIG. 51
Recurrence of the left inferior laryngeal nerve with right aortic arch and retro-esophageal left subclavian artery.

The tumors are usually accessible through a cervical incision, since they are small, rarely descend far, and usually possess a recognizable pedicle from a thyroid artery. Black (1953) emphasizes that thoracotomy is rarely necessary (2 of 102 cases of hyperparathyroidism in his series).

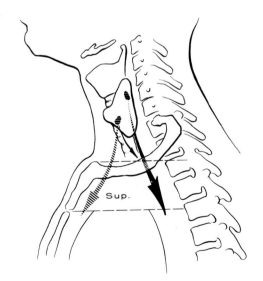

Sup.

FIG. 52
Paths of developmental migration, or adult displacement, of parathyroid adenomas. (From Black, in Cooper, 1971.)

THYMUS

That the thymus is partly a cervical organ is most apparent in the newborn (Fig. 53). Its embryonic association with the parathyroid and thyroid glands is indicated by the frequent discovery of thymic tissue in or about those structures (Fig. 54), and the frequent location of a parathyroid gland within the substance of the thymus. Thus, even in the adult, portions of the thymus gland may be located in the neck, where branches from the inferior thyroid artery lead into the gland.

The lower limit of the gland, in the adult, varies from the first intercostal space to the level of the xiphoid process, with most thymus glands extending to a level between the third and fourth costal cartilages (Bell *et al.,* 1954). The

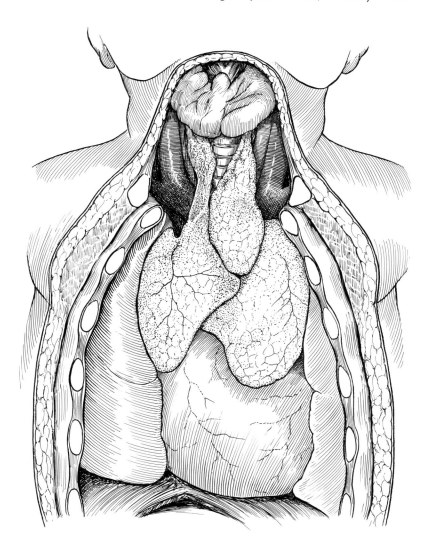

FIG. 53
The thymus in a newborn. (After Kiss and Szentagothai, 1964.)

bilobed structure of the gland remains evident in the adult. The lobes can generally be easily separated in the midline, where the only major vascular connection is the thymic vein draining both lobes and terminating in the left brachiocephalic vein (Fig. 56). Other veins drain laterally and superiorly into the inferior thyroid veins. The major arterial supply enters laterally, being derived most frequently from the internal thoracic arteries (Bell *et al.*, 1954). Bell and his colleagues and Sloan (1943) (Fig. 55) describe a variable supply from the inferior thyroid artery and other branches of the subclavian artery.

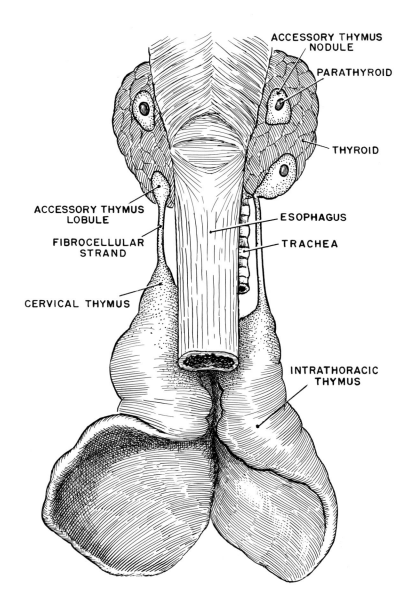

FIG. 54
Thymic rests. (After Groschuff, 1900, and Romanes, 1964.)

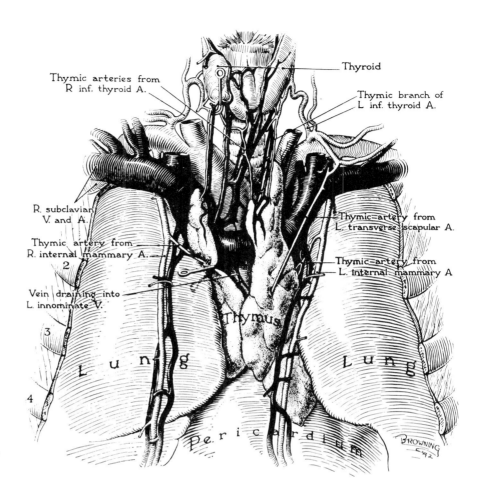

Thyroid

Thymic arteries from
R. inf. thyroid A.

Thymic branch of
L. inf. thyroid A.

R. subclavian
V. and A.

Thymic artery from
L. transverse scapular A.

Thymic artery from
R. internal mammary A.

Thymic artery from
L. internal mammary A.

2

Vein draining into
L. innominate V.

Thymus

3

Lung

Lung

4

Pericardium

BROWNING
'42

FIG. 55
Vascular supply of the thymus. (From Sloan, 1943.)

The possibility of exposing the gland by extrapleural posterior mediastinotomy [sic!] (Lilienthal, 1925) is of historical interest. Currently the approach most generally used is a midsternal incision (Fig. 56, and p. 95). Crile (1966) has brought back the suprasternal approach of Crotti. He makes a low collar incision deepened through the infrahyoid muscles and fascia, and searches for the upper part of the thymus in the low cervical and substernal fat. The gland is whiter than the fat, smooth and firm, and often shows a fibrous or vascular band extending to the thyroid gland. Carlens (1967), using this approach, often adds mediastinoscopy to ensure that all of the thymus has been removed.

REFERENCES

Adams, H. D.: Transthoracic thyroidectomy. J. Thor. Surg. 19:741–750, 1950.

Anson, B. J.: An Atlas of Human Anatomy. Philadelphia, W. B. Saunders, 1950.

Bahnson, H. T., and Blalock, A.: Aortic vascular rings encountered in the surgical treatment of congenital pulmonic stenosis. Ann. Surg. 131:356–362, 1950.

Bell, R. H., Knapp, B. I., Anson, B. J., and Laeson, S. J.: Form, size, blood-supply and relations of the adult thymus. Quart. Bull. Northw. Univ. Med. Sch. 28:156–164, 1954.

Black, B. M.: Hyperparathyroidism. Springfield, Charles C Thomas, 1953.

Black, B. M.: Hyperparathyroidism. Chapter 12 in The Craft of Surgery, Cooper, P., Ed., 2nd ed. Vol. 1. Boston, Little, Brown, 1971.

Bugden, W. F., Straehley, C. J., Jr., and Ikins, P. M.: Two cases of posterior mediastinal goiter and their management. Surgery 45:941–944, 1959.

Carlens, E., Johansson, L., and Olsson, P.: La médiastinoscopie auxiliaire de la thymectomie par voie cervicale. Bronches 17:408–410, 1967.

Crile, G., Jr.: Thymectomy through the neck. Surgery 59:213–215, 1966.

Falor, W. H., Kelly, T. R., and Krabill, W. S.: Intrathoracic goiter. Ann. Surg. 142:238–247, 1955.

Groschuff, K.: Ueber das Vorkommen eines Thymussegmentes der vierten Kiementasche beim Menschen. Anat. Anz. 17:161–170, 1900.

Henle, J.: Handbuch des systematischen Anatomie des Menschen. Vol. 3, Handbuch der Gefässlehre. Braunschweig, Friedrich Vieweg und Sohn, 1868.

Holzapfel, G.: Ungewöhnlicher Ursprung und Verlauf der Arteria Subclavia Dextra. Anat. Hefte 12:369–526, 1899.

Kiss, F., and Szentágothai, J.: Atlas of Human Anatomy, 17th ed. Vol. 2. Oxford, Pergamon Press, 1964.

Lahey, F. H., and Swinton, N. W.: Intrathoracic goiter. Surg. Gynec. Obstet. 59:627–637, 1934.

Lilienthal, H.: Thoracic Surgery. Philadelphia. Saunders, 1925.

Quain, R.: The Anatomy of the Arteries of the Human Body. London, Taylor and Walton, 1844.

Randolph, J., Grunt, J. A., and Vawter, G. F.: The medical and surgical aspects of intratracheal goiter. New Eng. J. Med. 268:457–461, 1963.

Romanes, G. J., Ed.: Cunningham's Textbook of Anatomy, 10th ed. London, Oxford, 1964.

Schaeffer, J. P., Ed.: Morris' Human Anatomy, 11th ed. New York, Blakiston, 1953.

Sloan, H. E., Jr.: The thymus in myasthenia gravis. With observations on the normal anatomy and histology of the thymus. Surgery 13:154–174, 1943.

Sweet, R. H.: Intrathoracic goiter located in the posterior mediastinum. Surg. Gynec. Obstet. 89:57–66, 1949.

Tamoney, H. J.: Surgery for thyroid cancer. Amer. J. Surg. 119:699–701, 1970.

SECTION 3

The Heart and Pericardium

MEdiAN STERNOTOMY

EXPOSURE

Median sternotomy with lateral retraction of the halves of the sternum is the most versatile incision for cardiac surgery, offering good exposure of all the chambers and valves of the heart. It is also an excellent approach for operations on the intrathoracic trachea, thymus, and great vessels of the superior mediastinum.

As illustrated in the upper insert of Figure 56, the skin is incised in the midline from the upper border of the manubrium to a point well below the xiphoid. Careful positioning of the incision in the exact midline minimizes bleeding and avoids fibers of the pectoralis major as they arise from the sternum. The inferior extension allows wide sternal retraction. Superiorly, the incision passes through the suprasternal space of Burns, where there may be a large communication between the two anterior jugular veins. The interclavicular ligament is divided on the upper border of the sternum. Below, the incision divides the linea alba and enters the preperitoneal fat through the transversalis fascia.

In the older Duval-Barasty exposure, the peritoneum was opened, and the diaphragm was split to the hepatic coronary ligament (Lilienthal, 1925). As splitting of the sternum commences above, anterior traction on the bone lifts it from the underlying areolar tissue binding the pleurae and pericar-

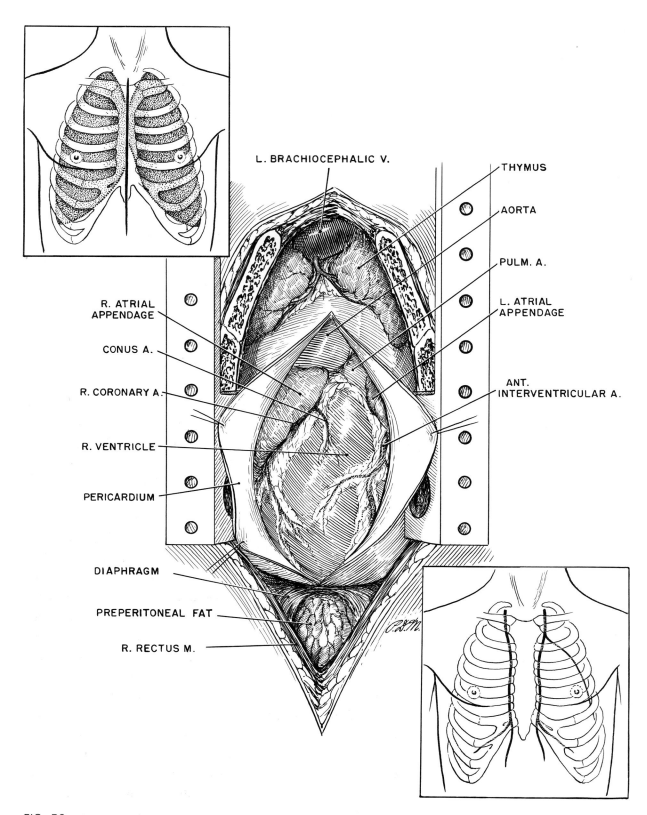

L. BRACHIOCEPHALIC V.

THYMUS

AORTA

PULM. A.

L. ATRIAL APPENDAGE

ANT. INTERVENTRICULAR A.

R. ATRIAL APPENDAGE

CONUS A.

R. CORONARY A.

R. VENTRICLE

PERICARDIUM

DIAPHRAGM

PREPERITONEAL FAT

R. RECTUS M.

FIG. 56
Median sternotomy. The lower insert shows an anomalous lateral costal artery.

dium to the sternum. The so-called pericardiacosternal ligaments are hardly discernible as separate structures. The periosteum and connective tissue may be highly vascular in cyanotic congenital heart disease. Sternal retraction is facilitated by partial division of the xiphoid origins of the diaphragm on either side of the midline.

The configuration of the thorax is that of a truncated cone flattened somewhat in the anteroposterior dimension. When the sternum is retracted, the greatest width is obtained in the lower portion. The retractor blades should always be placed at the lower third of the sternum to ensure maximum exposure without too wide a separation of the halves of the manubrium. Excessive separation of the upper portion of the incision stretches the brachial plexus over the first rib and has been responsible for nerve injury in some instances.

The course of the internal thoracic arteries is shown about 1.5 cm to either side of the sternum in the lower insert of Figure 56. A lateral costal artery, shown arising from the left internal thoracic artery, may be found on one side in 28 per cent and on both sides in 5 per cent (Kropp, 1951).

The pleurae meet in the upper part of the exposure, often somewhat to the right or left of the midline. The line of divergence of the left pleura is shown in the upper insert, where its mean deviation from the sternal border is only 2 mm in the fifth intercostal space (Woodburne, 1947). This leaves no more than about a square centimeter to constitute the 'bare area of the pericardium' uncovered by pleura to the left of the sternum. Figure 57 illustrates the range of deviation of the anterior lines of pleural reflection.

VIEWS OF PERICARDIUM, THYMUS, HEART, AND MAJOR VESSELS

In the adult the medial borders of the pleurae are seen inferior to and beneath the small thymus. The pericardium is easily exposed through the relatively avascular tissue separating the two pleurae and the two lobes of the thymus. The veins of the thymus unite as a short single thymic vein which travels between the lobes to intercept the left brachiocephalic vein. The principal arterial supply of the thymus enters from the lateral aspect of each lobe, usually from the internal

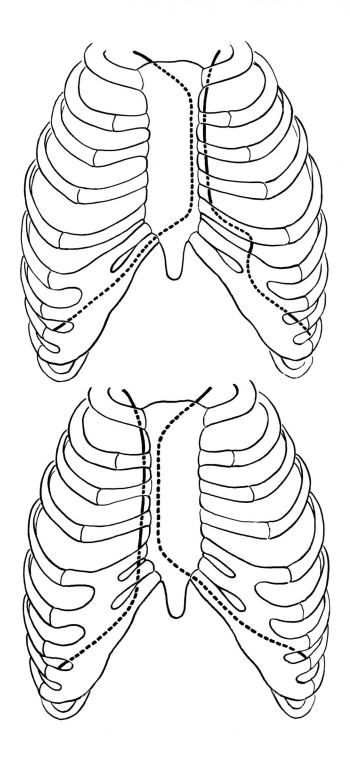

FIG. 57
Maximal deviation of anterior lines of pleural reflection. (After Tanja, 1891.)

thoracic arteries (Fig. 55). In the child the gland is very large, often hiding the anterior aspect of the pleural borders and much of the pericardium (Fig. 53). After puberty, the thymus becomes progressively smaller. Even in the child, the plane between the lobes is usually readily found and the lobes are easily parted. The thymus is further considered on page 85.

Congenital defects of the pericardium are almost invariably left sided (Hollinshead, 1956), with continuity of the left pleural and the pericardial cavity. Sunderland and Wright-Smith (1944) described two cases in which large anterior portions of pericardium were lacking.

The heart is exposed by incising the pericardium from its aortic reflection to the diaphragm. Relaxing incisions may be made in the pericardium above the tendinous portion of the diaphragm, from the midline toward the inferior vena cava on the right and toward the cardiac apex on the left (see Fig. 58).

Covering the right aspect of the base of the aorta is the right atrial appendage. A few avascular adhesions occasionally bind the appendage to the aorta. The right atrium is thin and fragile anterior to the crista terminalis. This area is distinguished by its darker color and softness to palpation as compared with the atrial wall posteriorly.

The atrioventricular groove is marked by fat beneath the visceral pericardium. In this fat lies the right coronary artery. The conus branch crosses the right ventricular outflow tract approximately at the line of the crista supraventricularis of the right ventricle. Schlesinger et al. (1949) state that the conus artery is a separate and third coronary artery in 50 per cent of persons, originating from the same sinus as the right coronary artery. It extends to the left coronary artery in the ring of Vieussens (James, 1961). Gerbode et al. (1962) proposed that the right ventricle be opened by a low transverse incision to preserve major muscle bundles (see Fig. 68). This incision also avoids injury to the conus artery or to an anomalous anterior interventricular artery arising from the right coronary artery (see Fig. 73).

Figure 58 illustrates the lines of reflection of the pericardium, a knowledge of which is helpful in isolating the major vessels. Note the lack of communication between the transverse and oblique sinuses, and between the oblique sinus and the right pericardial gutter. The venae cavae are

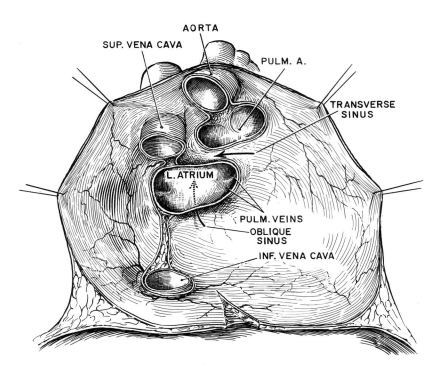

attached at their posterior surfaces, their anterior surfaces lying free in the pericardial cavity. If the left brachiocephalic vein is small, the presence of a left superior vena cava should be suspected (see Fig. 65). The pulmonary veins vary in length. They may enter the pericardial cavity individually, having a short segment free anteriorly within the cavity (see Fig. 97), but this is quite variable (p. 197). At times the two veins of one side may join before they enter the pericardial cavity. The proximal aorta and the main pulmonary artery are bound together by loose connective tissue and by the common covering of visceral pericardium. The two vessels thus form a single mass lying free within the transverse sinus. The nerves and lymphatics of the heart are intimately associated with both vessels and are subject to injury during dissection (see Figs. 86 and 87).

Notice the vascular pattern of the posterior pericardium in Figure 58. The rather tiny vessels have been injected with India ink to illustrate their communication with the vasa vasorum of the great vessels at the lines of pericardial reflection. These vasa vasorum, especially about the pulmonary veins, communicate with branches of the coronary arteries. This is elaborated on in the discussion of the coronary circulation (Chapter 16).

REFERENCES

Gerbode, F., Ross, J. K., March, H. W., Osborn, J. J., and Kerth, W. J.: Transverse ventriculotomy. Bull. Soc. Int. Chir. 21:345–353, 1962.

Hollinshead, W. H.: Anatomy for Surgeons. Vol. 2, The Thorax, Abdomen, and Pelvis. New York, Hoeber, 1956.

Hudson, C. L., Moritz, A. R., and Wearn, J. T.: The extracardiac anastomoses of the coronary arteries. J. Exp. Med. 56:919–925, 1932.

James, T. N.: Anatomy of the Coronary Arteries. New York, Hoeber, 1961.

Kropp, B. N.: The lateral costal branch of the internal mammary artery. J. Thor. Surg. 21:421–425, 1951.

Lilienthal, H.: Thoracic Surgery. Philadelphia, W. B. Saunders, 1925.

Schlesinger, M. J., Zoll, P. M., and Wessler, S.: The conus artery. A third coronary artery. Amer. Heart J. 38:823–836, 1949.

Sunderland, S., and Wright-Smith, R. J.: Congenital pericardial defects. Brit. Heart J. 6:167–175, 1944.

Tanja, T.: Über die Grenzen der Pleurahöhlen bei den Primaten und bei einigen anderen Säugethieren. Morph. Jahrb. 17:145–197, 1891.

Woodburne, R. T.: The costomediastinal border of the left pleura in the precordial area. Anat. Rec. 97:197–210, 1947.

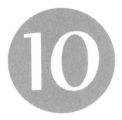

Right-sided approach to the atria; mitral-valve replacement

PERICARDIAL ATTACHMENT TO THE GREAT VEINS

The right side of the heart may be approached by median sternotomy or right anterolateral thoracotomy. The heart is rotated upward and to the left in Figure 59 A. The superior vena cava enters the pericardium to the right of the aorta. Anteriorly the vena cava lies free within the pericardium. Posteriorly it is attached by pericardial reflections to the left atrium, right pulmonary artery, and the posterior and lateral parietal pericardium. Between the azygos vein above and the atria below, a cul-de-sac of pericardium protrudes from the right lateral aspect, partially beneath the vena cava, separating it from the pulmonary artery (see Fig. 58).

The azygos vein joins the posterior aspect of the superior vena cava after sweeping forward above the right pulmonary artery. Notice the position of the tape in Figure 59 A. The vena cava has been encircled directly anterior to the pulmonary artery, avoiding trauma to the azygos vein above and the area of the sinu-atrial node below. Division of pericardial attachments in this area is usually bloodless and the resulting mobility enables the operator to visualize the superior aspect of the left atrium beneath the vena cava. The right pulmonary

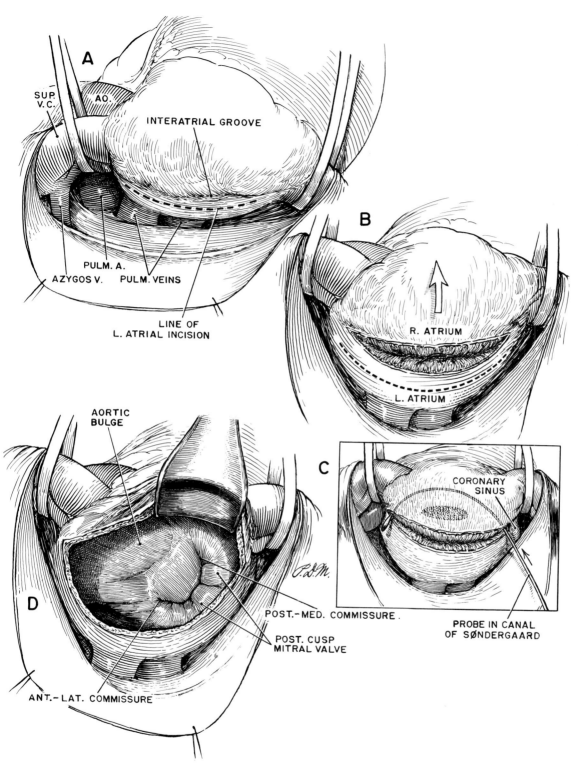

FIG. 59
Right-sided exposure of the atria and the mitral valve through median sternotomy.

veins are seen entering the lateral wall of the left atrium, posterior to the interatrial groove. The pericardial attachments of the inferior vena cava have been divided posteriorly and a tape has been passed around the vena cava. This is easily accomplished in most instances since, as seen in Figure 58, the inferior vena cava is almost totally intrapericardial just above the diaphragm, with the reflection lying posterior and lateral.

MITRAL-VALVE REPLACEMENT

The dotted lines of Figure 59 A and B indicate the position of an incision in the left atrium commonly used for exposure of the mitral valve. This incision is placed in the left atrial wall between the right pulmonary veins and the interatrial groove. Excellent exposure of the interior of the left atrium can be obtained. If the left atrium is small and tucked beneath the right atrium, the interatrial groove may be dissected as illustrated in Figure 59 B. The epicardium has been sharply divided and the right atrium pushed upward and medially. A few small veins may be encountered. The interatrial groove contains loose fibro-areolar tissue and extends circumferentially around the area of the true septum in the 'canal of Søndergaard.' Søndergaard and his colleagues (1955) used this anatomical feature in closing atrial septal defects. A heavy ligature was passed about the defect in a manner similar to passage of the probe in Figure 59 C. The ligature was tied to obliterate the defect. The probe in Figure 59 C was introduced into the interatrial groove in the dimple between the coronary sinus, inferior vena cava, and right atrial wall as described by Wilson *et al.* (1958).

In Figure 59 D the incision previously outlined has been opened. The mitral valve is exposed. The orifices of the pulmonary veins are obscured by the posterior edge of the left atrium. The bulge cephalad to the major mitral cusp is caused by the non-coronary sinus of the aorta. The orifice of the left atrial appendage is seen posterior and cephalad to the mitral valve. The anterior and posterior cusps of the mitral valve are readily identified. A small cusplike fold may often be seen at the commissures. Such accessory cusps have little surgical significance.

THE CARDIAC SKELETON AND
ATRIOVENTRICULAR PERIMETER

The fibrous 'cardiac skeleton' is shown in Figure 60. This configuration has been described by Zimmerman and Bailey (1962), and it has been confirmed by our dissections. The skeleton is composed of an anulus, or fibrous ring, at the periphery of each cardiac valve, with areas of continuity between the four rings. The anulus of the pulmonic valve forms a continuous tri-arched buttress in the vessel wall at the base of the three cusps. It is only about 1 mm thick, but it is tough. This anulus is connected to the rest of the skeleton by the poorly defined 'conus ligament,' attaching the pulmonic to the aortic walls. The aortic anulus, a similar tri-arched structure, is 1.5 to 2 mm thick. It is connected to the atrioventricular valve rings at the small left and the larger right fibrous trigone. The right trigone gives passage to the atrioventricular bundle (Fig. 75), which may here be impinged on by too deep positioning of sutures in procedures for replacement of the aortic or tricuspid valve.

The rings of the atrioventricular valves are tenuous fibrous structures, the external limit of which is hard to distinguish from the ventricular muscle arising from them. At their outer

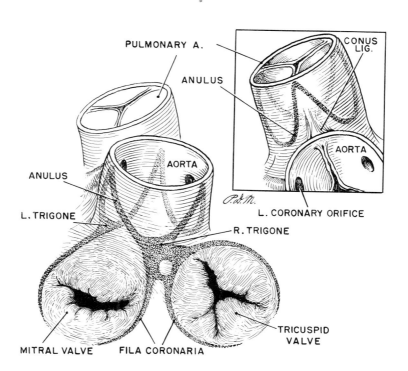

FIG. 60
The skeleton of the heart. (After Zimmerman and Bailey, 1962.)

edges lie the right main and the left circumflex coronary artery, the coronary sinus, and the small cardiac vein (Fig. 61). In their concavities course the thin rounded bands termed the fila coronaria (Fig. 60). The fila extend from the left and right trigones. Zimmerman and Bailey (1962) have emphasized the delicacy of these structures. Henle (1868) had already complained that artists pictured them too heavily and had represented them as rings, whereas they often encompassed only one-sixth of the circumference of the valves. He stated that the fila may be absent; this is less likely in the mitral valve. Although the fila of the mitral valve are stronger than the fila of the tricuspid, they are less than 1 mm thick.

These fibrous bands are of importance to the cardiac surgeon since they constitute the toughest portion of the anulus of the atrioventricular valves. Indeed, in one-fourth to one-third of the circumference where the fila are absent, the valve cusp itself preserves the endocardial integrity. When the posterior cusp of the mitral valve is totally resected, dehiscence of the fatty tissue of the atrioventricular groove may occur with massive bleeding. The coronary sinus

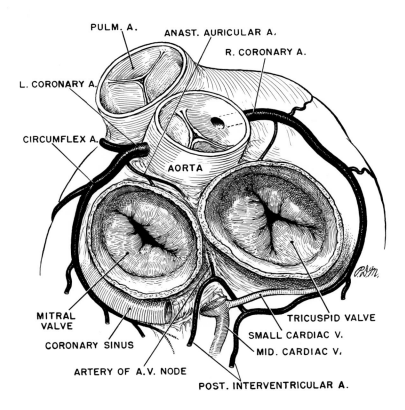

FIG. 61
Structures in the atrioventricular perimeter.

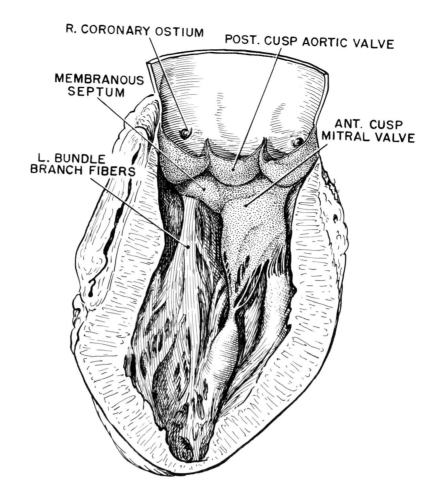

R. CORONARY OSTIUM

POST. CUSP AORTIC VALVE

MEMBRANOUS SEPTUM

ANT. CUSP MITRAL VALVE

L. BUNDLE BRANCH FIBERS

FIG. 62
Interior of the left ventricle, showing continuity of aortic wall with anterior cusp of mitral valve, and the membranous interventricular septum. (After Spalteholz, 1954.)

and circumflex coronary artery are also within dangerous reach. Most surgeons therefore prefer to leave a goodly portion of the relatively tough cusp posteriorly to provide firm fixation for the sutures in mitral valve replacement.

An additional hazard in mitral valve surgery is the distortion of the aortic valve which may result from excessive traction by sutures of the anterior mitral cusp. More commonly, mitral distortion may be produced by aortic valve replacement. These potential problems stem from the continuity of the anterior cusp of the mitral valve and the posterior wall of the aorta (Fig. 62).

The circumferences of the heart valves at various ages are shown in Figure 63. Saphir (1953) gives the averages for the adult as follows: mitral, 10 cm; aortic, 7.5 cm; pulmonic, 8.5 cm; tricuspid, 12 cm.

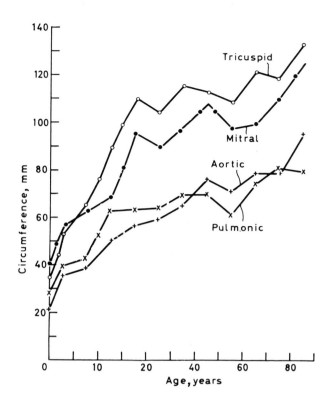

FIG. 63
Circumferences of the heart valves, showing modification with age. (Adapted from Kirch, 1921, and Roessle and Roulet, 1932.)

References

Henle, J.: Handbuch des systematischen Anatomie des Menschen. Vol. 3. Handbuch der Gefässlehre. Braunschweig, Friedrich Vieweg und Sohn, 1868.

Kirch, E.: Über gesetzmässige Verschiebungen der inneren Grössenverhältnisse des normalen und pathologisch veränderten menschlichen Herzens. Zschr. f. Angewandte Anat. u. Konstit. 7:235–384, 1921.

Roessle, R., and Roulet, F.: Mass und Zahl in der Pathologie. Berlin, Springer, 1932.

Saphir, O.: Weights and Measurements of Heart. P. 969 *in* Pathology of the Heart, Gould, S. E., Ed. Springfield, Charles C Thomas, 1953.

Sondergaard, T., Gøtzsche, H., Ottosen, P., and Schultz, J.: Surgical closure of interatrial septal defects by circumclusion. Acta Chir. Scand. 109:188–196, 1955.

Spalteholz, W.: Hand-Atlas of Human Anatomy, 15th ed. Revised by Spanner, R. Vol II, Part II. Vascular System, Viscera, Nervous System, Sense Organs. Boston, Little, Brown, 1954.

Wilson, H. E., Cardozo, R. H., Kee, J. L., and Siebel, E. K.: Closure of interatrial secundum defects: simplified by utilization of previously undescribed anatomic feature. Amer. Surg. 24: 439–451, 1958.

Zimmerman, J., and Bailey, C. P.: The surgical significance of the fibrous skeleton of the heart. J. Thorac. Cardiovasc. Surg. 44:701–712, 1962.

EXPOSURE OF MITRAL VALVE FROM THE LEFT; THE AORTIC VALVE

INTERIOR OF LEFT ATRIUM AND VENTRICLE

In Figure 64 A, the heart has been approached by posterolateral thoracotomy, and it is viewed from the left. The pericardium has been turned back except for a narrow strip over which course the phrenic nerve and pericardiacophrenic artery and veins. This neurovascular bundle is best left attached to the pericardium for protection against damage by stretching. The proposed left atrial incision is shown. Its crescentic outline allows an opening of maximal size without encroachment on the atrioventricular groove below or medially. The left atrial wall is delicate, particularly in elderly persons and in the presence of pulmonary venous hypertension.

In Figure 64 B, the atrium has been opened, exposing the mitral valve. The anterior (major) and posterior (minor) cusps are thrown into folds in the closed position and it appears that smaller accessory leaflets occupy the commissures of the valve.

In Figure 64 C, the left ventricle has been opened. It is evident why the anterior mitral cusp is frequently called the mitral 'curtain.' It spreads as a baffle, forming the postero-

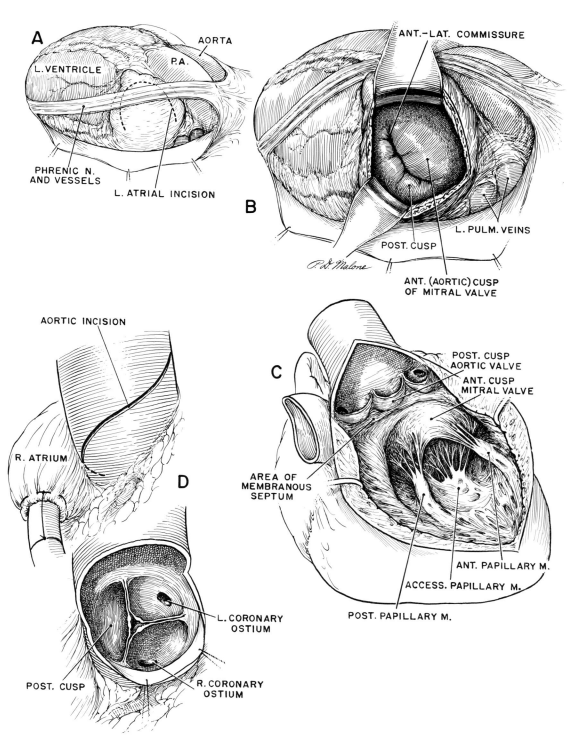

A

L. VENTRICLE

AORTA

P.A.

PHRENIC N.
AND VESSELS

L. ATRIAL INCISION

B

ANT.-LAT. COMMISSURE

L. PULM. VEINS

POST. CUSP

P. D. Malone

ANT. (AORTIC) CUSP
OF MITRAL VALVE

AORTIC INCISION

R. ATRIUM

D

POST. CUSP

L. CORONARY
OSTIUM

R. CORONARY
OSTIUM

C

POST. CUSP
AORTIC VALVE

ANT. CUSP
MITRAL VALVE

AREA OF
MEMBRANOUS
SEPTUM

ANT. PAPILLARY M.

ACCESS. PAPILLARY M.

POST. PAPILLARY M.

FIG. 64
Interior of the left atrium and ventricle. A, B. Exposure of mitral valve as by left thoracotomy. C. View by anatomic dissection. D. Exposure of aortic valve as by median sternotomy.

medial boundary of the left ventricular outflow tract. The base of this cusp is continuous with the aortic base between the middle of the left coronary cusp and the middle of the non-coronary cusp (see also Fig. 62). This relationship serves to distinguish the normal state from the distortions that may occur in certain forms of congenital heart disease (double-outlet right ventricle) in which the aorta is displaced toward the right ventricle and away from the mitral valve. Perforation of the major mitral cusp may result from overzealous removal of calcium during surgery for calcific aortic stenosis. Too-deep placement of sutures for an aortic-valve prosthesis may result in upward displacement of the major cusp with consequent mitral insufficiency.

Each of the two papillary muscles gives origin to numerous chordae tendineae which pass to both cusps. The commissures thus lie in the arms of chordae from both muscles. Fusion of the commissures in mitral stenosis may be compounded by shortening, fusion, and thickening of the chordae, to form subvalvular obstruction. The anterior papillary muscle receives arteries from both the left anterior interventricular and the circumflex coronary artery. The posterior papillary muscle is almost totally dependent on either the circumflex or the distal right coronary artery. Infarction or fibrosis of the posterior muscle is most frequently responsible for papillary muscle dysfunction causing mitral insufficiency in coronary artery disease.

The left ventricular myocardium is thicker than the right, averaging 8 to 10 mm, but trabeculation of the left ventricular cavity is less marked. Overlapping layers of ventricular myocardium contribute to the twisting and squeezing motion of contraction which empties the ventricle (see Fig. 68). A small dimple at the apex of the left ventricle is readily palpable in most hearts. This thin zone most devoid of vital parts is frequently used for the insertion of a catheter for decompression of the left ventricle during open cardiac surgery.

EXPOSURE OF THE AORTIC VALVE

Figure 64 D shows a useful incision for exposure of the aortic valve. The lower portion of the incision has been carried into the sinus of the non-coronary cusp. This opens the aortic base while the incision remains accessible should there be bleeding after closure. The incision may be safely carried further if necessary for better exposure, transecting the arched fibrous anulus. The atrioventricular bundle lies between the non-coronary (posterior) cusp and the right coronary cusp (Fig. 75), and should not be injured by this incision.

The cusps of the aortic valve are not of equal size. The non-coronary cusp is larger than either the right or the left. The cusps are normally very thin and delicate structures. There is some thickening at their free edges, accentuated at the mid-point as the nodule. In perhaps as many as 20 per cent there may be tiny fenestrations of the cusps near the free edge close to the commissural attachments. These are usually of no functional importance, but aortic insufficiency has occasionally resulted.

ANOMALOUS LEFT SUPERIOR VENA CAVA AND RETRO-AORTIC LEFT BRACHIOCEPHALIC VEIN

In anterior left cardiac exposures, one may encounter an anomalous left superior vena cava or other variations of the left brachiocephalic vein. The embryonic left superior vena cava is ordinarily evanescent, leaving behind the oblique ligament of the left atrium, attached to the coronary sinus and containing the small oblique vein (of Marshall) entering the sinus (see Fig. 83). The left superior vena cava (Fig. 65) persists in about 0.5 per cent (Adachi, 1933). In such cases, the right brachiocephalic vein usually continues its course as the superior vena cava, receiving a small connection from the left. The condition may therefore also be called doubling of the superior vena cava. More rarely the right superior vena cava is absent, the persistent left vena cava receiving the right brachiocephalic vein (Edwards, 1968).

As on the right, the left superior vena cava receives the left internal jugular and subclavian veins, as well as the left superior intercostal vein which drains a variable part of the left azygos, or hemiazygos system. The large trunk thus formed replaces the usually small oblique vein, and also terminates in the coronary sinus, which then becomes a very wide vessel.

5

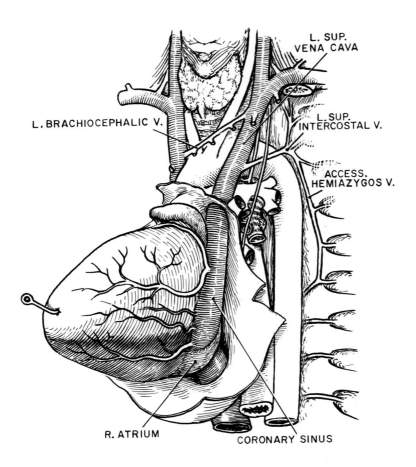

FIG. 65
Anomalous left superior vena cava.
(After Adachi, 1933.)

As previously noted, a small left brachiocephalic vein alerts one to the likelihood of a left superior vena cava. A left superior vena cava must be dealt with in controlling venous return in open heart surgery. The large vessel is also in the field in operations on a patent ductus arteriosus or on the left lung. The persistent left superior vena cava may open into the left atrium when there is concomitant atresia of the right atrial ostium of the coronary sinus and atrial septal defect. It may be involved in anomalous pulmonary venous drainage (Edwards *et al.*, 1954).

Woodburne (1951) reported a case of doubling of the superior vena cava, each vessel receiving its own azygos vein, associated with a right aortic arch.

Adachi (1933) illustrated two rare situations in which, until the pericardium was opened, a left superior vena cava was suspected because of a posterior position of the left brachiocephalic vein (Fig. 66). This vein coursed to its right superior caval termination in one case behind the ascending

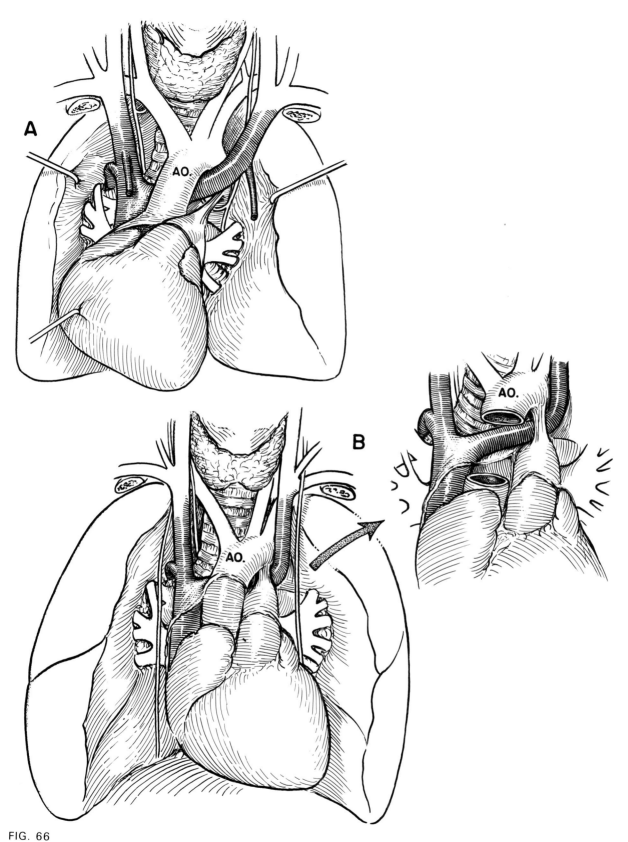

FIG. 66
Two examples of retro-aortic left brachiocephalic vein: one anterior (A) and one posterior (B) to the ligamentum arteriosum. (After Adachi, 1933.)

aorta and in front of the ligamentum arteriosum, and in the other case behind both the arch of the aorta and the ligamentum arteriosum.

REFERENCES

Adachi, B.: Das Venensystem der Japaner. Tokyo, Kenkyusha, 1933.

Edwards, J. E.: Congenital Malformations of the Heart and Great Vessels. Chapter 9 *in* Pathology of the Heart, Gould, S. E., Ed., 3rd ed. Springfield, Charles C Thomas, 1968.

Edwards, J. E., Dry, T. J., Parker, R. L., Burchell, H. D., Wood, E. H., and Bulbulian, A. H.: An Atlas of Congenital Anomalies of the Heart and Great Vessels. Springfield, Charles C Thomas, 1954.

Woodburne, R. T.: A case of right aortic arch and associated venous anomalies. Anat. Rec. 111:617–627, 1951.

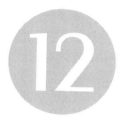

Right Atrium and Ventricle

INTERIOR OF THE RIGHT ATRIUM AND VENTRICLE

In Figure 67 A the lateral wall of the right atrium has been opened widely. The 'interatrial septum' forms the posterior and medial walls of the right atrium. As shown in Figure 59, a common septum truly exists only in the area of the fossa ovalis and the surrounding anulus fossae ovalis. The remainder of the interatrial septum superiorly includes the muscle and endocardium from each atrium and the intervening fatty tissue.

Inferiorly the endocardium of the right atrium covers the broad portion of the right fibrous trigone of the heart (see Fig. 60), from which originate the septal cusp of the tricuspid valve and the medial portion of the anterior cusp of the mitral valve. The fibrous trigone is not precisely horizontal but inclines inferiorly and posteriorly. Consequently the medial portion of the anterior mitral cusp originates a few millimeters above the origin of the septal tricuspid cusp. In this area only the fibrous trigone with its endothelial coverings and a few muscle fibers of the right atrial wall lie between the cavities of the right atrium and the left ventricle. Congenital 'cushion' defects may occur which allow communication between these two chambers.

The orifice of the coronary sinus is partially obscured by its endocardial valve (of Thebesius) as it enters the right

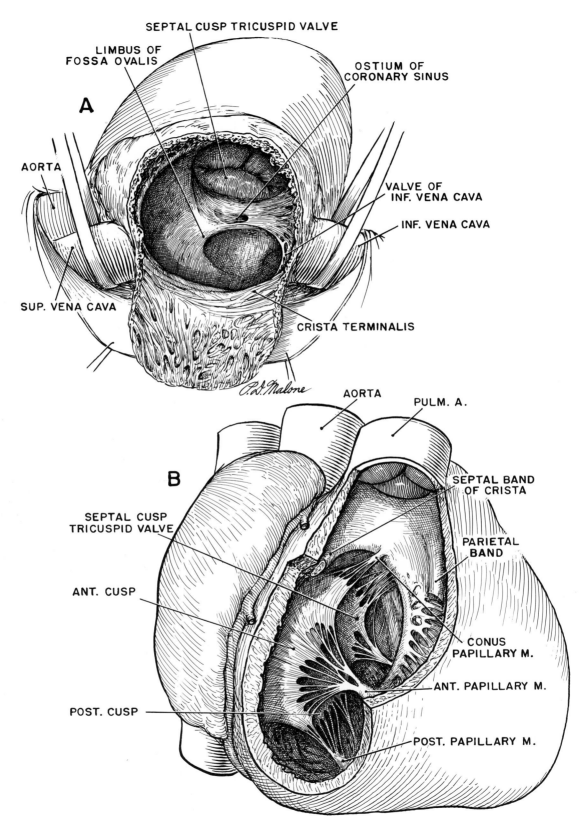

SEPTAL CUSP TRICUSPID VALVE

LIMBUS OF
FOSSA OVALIS

OSTIUM OF
CORONARY SINUS

A

AORTA

VALVE OF
INF. VENA CAVA

INF. VENA CAVA

SUP. VENA CAVA

CRISTA TERMINALIS

C. D. Malone

AORTA

PULM. A.

B

SEPTAL BAND
OF CRISTA

SEPTAL CUSP
TRICUSPID VALVE

PARIETAL
BAND

ANT. CUSP

CONUS
PAPILLARY M.

ANT. PAPILLARY M.

POST. CUSP

POST. PAPILLARY M.

FIG. 67
Interior of the right atrium (A) and right ventricle (B).

atrium between the inferior vena cava and the septal cusp of the tricuspid valve. The atrioventricular node lies between the orifice of the coronary sinus and the septal leaflet. Placement of sutures in this area during surgery on the tricuspid valve or in the repair of congenital anomalies may result in complete atrioventricular block (see Fig. 75).

Notice the smooth posterior portion of the right atrial wall, superior to the inferior vena cava and extending medially to the ostium of the coronary sinus. This portion of the wall corresponds to the primitive sinus venosus (see Fig. 69). The lateral and anterior atrial wall is covered by the musculi pectinati and corresponds to the embryonic atrium. The junction between the two portions of the atrium is marked by the crista terminalis, which sweeps from the front of the superior caval orifice to the front of the inferior vena cava. Externally the sulcus terminalis marks the course of the crista. The thicker, less fragile atrial wall posterior to the sulcus terminalis is frequently the site for placement of caval catheters for cardiopulmonary bypass because it holds the necessary sutures more securely.

Observe that the limbus fossae ovalis overhangs the upper border of the fossa ovalis slightly. A catheter passed upward through the inferior vena cava tends to catch on this ridge. With the limbus as a guide, the fossa ovalis can be punctured to determine pressures in and obtain blood samples from the left side of the heart during cardiac catheterization.

Inferiorly the caval orifice is partially covered by a usually fenestrated fold of endocardium. This is the valve of the inferior vena cava (Eustachian valve). It is variable in size and extent (see Fig. 70).

Figure 67 B depicts the interior of the right ventricle. Chordae tendineae attach the antero-septal commissure and adjacent cusps to the conus papillary muscle, a small structure which is an important surgical landmark for the conduction system (p. 135; Fig. 75 E). Accessory conus papillary muscles are also seen. The inferior-septal commissure is tethered to the posterior papillary muscle. The anterior papillary muscle supplies chordae to the antero-inferior commissure and adjacent areas of the anterior and posterior cusps. The chordae insert on the free edges of the cusps and on a variable portion of their ventricular surfaces. Thus complete surgical mobilization cannot be achieved by merely excising the free margins of the valve.

The trabeculae carneae are very prominent in the right ventricle. Wedging of the tip of a transvenous pacemaker catheter into the interstices of the trabeculae in the apex of the cavity secures the electrode against the endocardium. A constant trabecula is the moderator band (septomarginal trabecula), which courses as a ridge from near the base of the conus papillary muscle to the base of the anterior papillary muscle. It may lie free for a variable portion of its extent distally. Fibers of the right branch of the atrioventricular bundle travel in the moderator band.

The outflow tract of the right ventricle lies above and to the left of the tricuspid valve. Note its smooth walls. This is the infundibulum, or conus, of the right ventricle. It is bounded above by the pulmonary valve and below by a ridge, the crista supraventricularis, demarcating it from the trabeculated remainder of the right ventricle. The crista is a continuous structure, composed of a septal and a parietal band. Hypertrophy of the crista may produce significant obstruction of the right ventricular outflow tract.

THE VENTRICULAR MUSCULATURE

The ventricular musculature arises from the fibrous skeleton of the heart (see Fig. 60). By their contraction the upper portions of the various bundles act to constrict the ventricles, their lower spiralled parts shorten the long dimension of these chambers (Fig. 68). The muscles are responsible for competence of the atrioventricular valves, by acting as sphincters for the valve rings; through the continuity of their spiral portions with the papillary muscles they also prevent luxation of the valve leaflets into the atria.

It is evident that transverse or oblique incisions will do less damage than a vertical one to the musculature of either ventricle.

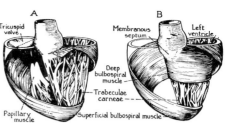

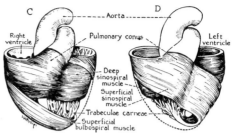

FIG. 68
The ventricular musculature.
A, B. The superficial and
deep bulbospiral muscles.
C, D. The superficial and
deep sinospiral muscles.
(From Rushmer, 1961,
after Robb and Robb,
1942.)

VALVULAR VARIATIONS AND NETWORKS IN THE RIGHT ATRIUM

The right atrium exhibits a wide range of normal variations in the valve of the inferior vena cava, valve of the coronary sinus, and the interatrial septum. Defects of the septum may be small and insignificant, or gross and distinctly abnormal. Interatrial septal defects less than 1 cm² in area do not cause equalization of the atrial pressures.

A brief reference to embryonic development of the heart may be helpful in explanation of these variations. Figure 69 A shows a well-developed valve of sinus venosus with right and left portions (labeled 'valvulae venosae'). The right valve of the sinus venosus gives rise to the valves of the inferior vena cava and the coronary sinus. The septum spurium and the cephalic part of the right valve persist as the crista terminalis. The interatrial septum is at first closed by the septum primum, which fuses with the atrioventricular canal endocardial cushion. Failure of this fusion results in a foramen primum ('interatrial foramen I') defect (see Fig. 75 D). A secondary resorption of the septum primum produces the foramen secundum ('interatrial foramen II'), which remains overlaid by the septum secundum ('septum II'), producing the foramen ovale. A lack of adequate development produces an interatrial septal defect of the 'secundum' type (see Fig. 71 C). Ordinarily the two components of the

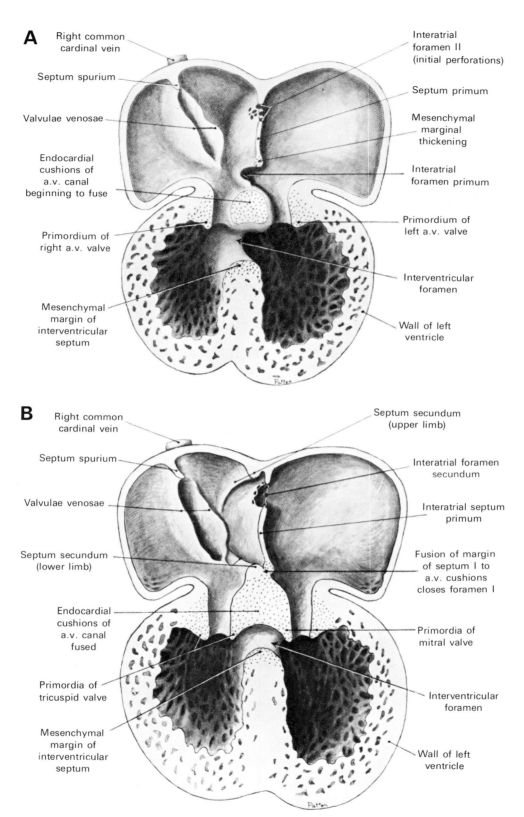

A

Right common cardinal vein

Septum spurium

Valvulae venosae

Endocardial cushions of a.v. canal beginning to fuse

Primordium of right a.v. valve

Mesenchymal margin of interventricular septum

Interatrial foramen II (initial perforations)

Septum primum

Mesenchymal marginal thickening

Interatrial foramen primum

Primordium of left a.v. valve

Interventricular foramen

Wall of left ventricle

B

Right common cardinal vein

Septum spurium

Valvulae venosae

Septum secundum (lower limb)

Endocardial cushions of a.v. canal fused

Primordia of tricuspid valve

Mesenchymal margin of interventricular septum

Septum secundum (upper limb)

Interatrial foramen secundum

Interatrial septum primum

Fusion of margin of septum I to a.v. cushions closes foramen I

Primordia of mitral valve

Interventricular foramen

Wall of left ventricle

FIG. 69
Embryology of the venous valves of the right atrium. A. Early stage. B. Later stage. (From Patten, 1960.)

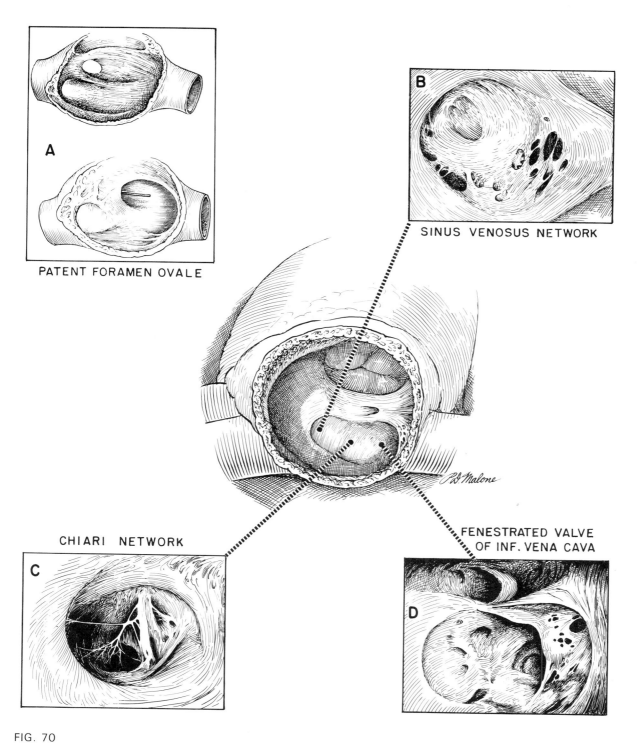

A

B

SINUS VENOSUS NETWORK

PATENT FORAMEN OVALE

P. D. Malone

CHIARI NETWORK

C

FENESTRATED VALVE
OF INF. VENA CAVA

D

FIG. 70

Valvular variations and networks in the right atrium. A. Patent foramen ovale, with 'pencil patency' above, and probe patency below. B. Sinus venosus network in the fossa ovalis. C. A Chiari network. D. Fenestrated valve of the inferior vena cava. (A after Wright et al., 1948; B after Edwards, 1968; C and D after Yater, 1929.)

interatrial septum fuse postnatally, leaving only a fossa at the site of the foramen ovale.

Figure 70 shows some of the normal variations resulting from deviations in the development described. Incomplete fusion of the septa at the fossa ovalis (Fig. 70 A) may produce an oblique patency. This may be of a size ('pencil patency') which, while ordinarily too small to be significant, may open obliquely to allow an embolus to pass from the right to the left side of the heart and give rise to paradoxical embolism. Thompson and Evans (1930) found 'pencil patency' in 6 per cent of autopsy specimens and 'probe patency' in 29 per cent. Remnants of the left valve of the sinus venosus may produce a trabecular network at the fossa ovalis (Fig. 70 B).

Figure 70 C illustrates a 'Chiari network,' which "may be defined as a network of fine or coarse fibers in the right atrium, its attachments extending from the region of the crista terminalis above, to the thebesian [coronary] and the eustachian [caval] valves, or even to the floor of the right atrium" (Edwards, 1968). The network is thought to represent incomplete absorption of the right valve of the sinus venosus or the septum spurium. Yater (1929) found a 3.3 per cent incidence at autopsy. The network may rarely be the site of thrombosis or lodgement of an embolus; it has no functional significance.

The valves of the inferior vena cava and of the coronary sinus vary in size. Fenestrations of these valves, as in Figure 70 D, are very frequent. It has happened that the surgeon has mistaken the fenestrations for an interatrial septal defect. In such instances the caval orifice has been sutured closed. Occasionally, during repair of secundum septal defects, a valve has been mistaken for the medial wall of the right atrium and the caval stream has been redirected into the left atrium.

REFERENCES

Edwards, J. E.: Congenital Malformations of the Heart and Great Vessels. Chapter 9 *in* Pathology of the Heart, Gould, S. E., Ed., 3rd ed. Springfield, Charles C Thomas, 1968.

Patten, B. M.: Persistent interatrial foramen primum. Amer. J. Anat. 107:271-280, 1960.

Robb, J. S., and Robb, R. C.: The normal heart. Anatomy and physiology of the structural units. Amer. Heart J. 23:455–467, 1942.

Rushmer, R. F.: Cardiovascular Dynamics. Philadelphia, W. B. Saunders, 1961.

Thompson, T., and Evans, W.: Paradoxical embolism. Quart. J. Med. 23:135–150, 1930.

Wright, R. R., Anson, B. J., and Cleveland, H. C.: The vestigial valves and the interatrial foramen of the adult human heart. Anat. Rec. 100:331–355, 1948.

Yater, W. M.: Variations and anomalies of the venous valves of the right atrium of the human heart. Arch. Path. 7:418–441, 1929.

congenital heart disease

THREE COMMON CARDIAC DEFECTS

Figure 71 A illustrates a congenital stenosis of the pulmonic valve and its exposure through the pulmonary trunk. Valve dimensions are considered on page 105 and in Figure 63.

Figure 71 B illustrates the tetralogy of Fallot, with a defect of the membranous part of the interventricular septum (see Fig. 62), the origin of the aorta overriding the defect ('dextroposition of the aorta'), subpulmonic stenosis, and hypertrophy of the right ventricle. The relationship of the defect and the hypertrophied crista supraventricularis to the atrioventricular conduction pathway makes that pathway vulnerable during surgical repair of the defect and excision of the hypertrophied crista, as is shown in Figure 75. The transverse incision shown in Figure 71 B is currently favored because its line is that of the conus coronary artery and of the major myocardial bundles (Fig. 68) (Gerbode et al., 1962). It may endanger the anterior interventricular or, more rarely, the entire left coronary artery, when these vessels originate from the right coronary artery, a condition that occurs with some frequency in congenitally abnormal hearts (see Fig. 73). The problem is even greater when the anomalous vessel is partly or entirely intramural (Fig. 72).

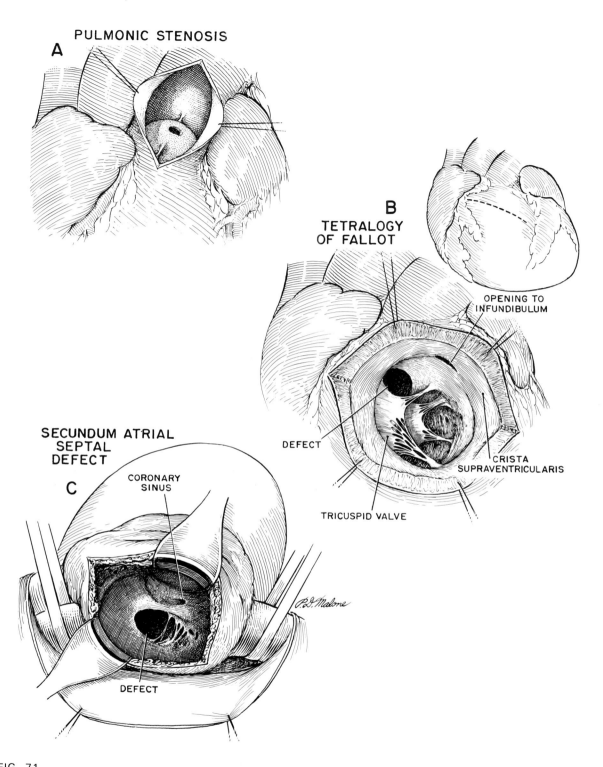

PULMONIC STENOSIS

A

B
**TETRALOGY
OF FALLOT**

OPENING TO
INFUNDIBULUM

DEFECT

CRISTA
SUPRAVENTRICULARIS

TRICUSPID VALVE

**SECUNDUM ATRIAL
SEPTAL
DEFECT**

C

CORONARY
SINUS

DEFECT

FIG. 71
*Three common congenital cardiac defects. A. Pulmonic stenosis. B. Tetralogy of Fallot. Insert shows line of
transverse incision in the right ventricle. C. Atrial septal defect of secundum type.*

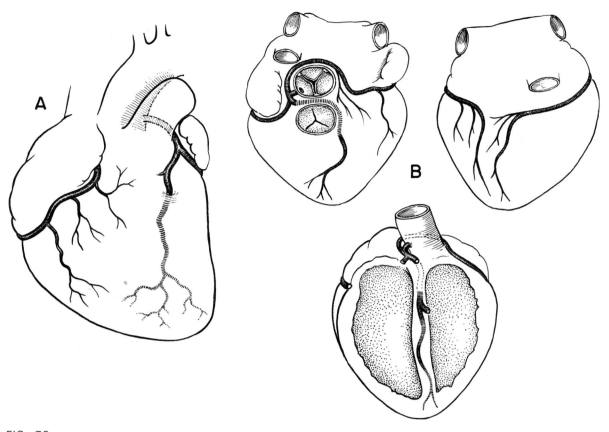

FIG. 72

Intramural course of coronary arteries. A. Intramural anterior interventricular artery. B. Single coronary artery with course of the anterior interventricular artery through the interventricular septum. (A, after Derrick et al., 1963; B, after Edwards et al., 1954.)

Figure 71 C shows an interatrial septal defect of the ostium secundum type. Its location, well behind the site of the atrioventricular node and bundle, makes repair relatively safe, in contrast to that of defects of the ostium primum variety (see Fig. 75).

MINOR VARIATIONS OF THE CORONARY ARTERIES

We may quickly dispose of three minor variations: (1) The conus artery may exist as a separate and third coronary artery, as mentioned on page 97. (2) A coronary artery may show early branching, as when the anterior interventricular and circumflex branches arise very close to the aortic sinus or with two separate ostia from the sinus; during open heart surgery, in such instances, a catheter placed in the left coronary artery may extend into the circumflex branch, blocking the orifice of the anterior interventricular branch. (3) Portions of the coronary arteries may course intramurally. Geiringer (1951) found that one of every five anterior interventricular arteries courses within the myocardium for all or part of its extent. This is pertinent to reconstruction of the coronary arteries, and also to the placement of cardiac incisions in congenital heart disease, such variations sometimes being associated with anomalous course of major coronary arteries (Fig. 72).

MAJOR VARIATIONS OF THE CORONARY ARTERIES

Two major categories of anomalous coronary arteries are known (Edwards, 1968). In the first (Fig. 73), the coronary system, although arising from the aorta, shows variations from the usual pattern or origin of the main coronary arteries or their branches. Origin of the anterior interventricular or of the circumflex artery from the right coronary (Fig. 73 E, F) is the most frequent major anomaly (Krumbhaar and Ehrich, 1938; Roberts and Loube, 1947; Edwards, 1968). In the second category one or both coronary arteries arise from or are connected to the pulmonary artery or the cardiac chambers (Fig. 74). The surgical significance of the first category is the possibility of accidental division of a coronary vessel. The second constitutes a pathologic entity by itself. Of greatest rarity is the origin of the coronary system from the brachiocephalic trunk, associated with major abnormalities of the heart and great vessels (Trevor, 1912; Bland et al., 1933).

Anomalous coronary arteries are rare except in patients with congenital heart disease. Of 31 cases of anomalous coronary arteries described by Roberts and Loube (1947), associated cardiac anomalies were present in 7. Major coronary anomalies were reported in 9 per cent of 183 patients with tetralogy of Fallot (combined reports of Kirklin et al., 1959, and Meng et al., 1965), and in 25 per cent of 135 hearts with complete transposition (Rowlatt, 1962).

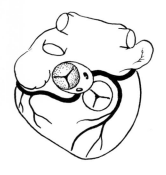
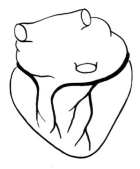

A BOTH CORONARY ARTERIES FROM
LEFT AORTIC SINUS

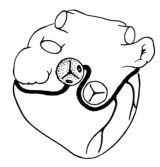
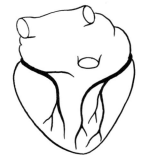

B LEFT CORONARY ARTERY
PASSING ANT. TO PULM. A.

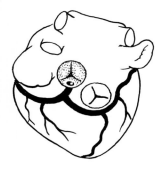
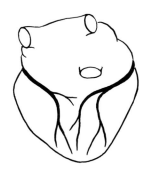

C SINGLE RIGHT CORONARY A.
WITH LEFT ARTERY PASSING
ANT. TO PULM. A.

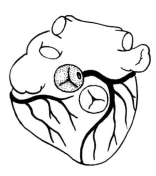
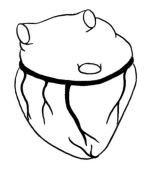

D SINGLE CORONARY A.
FROM LEFT AORTIC SINUS

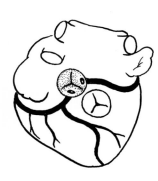
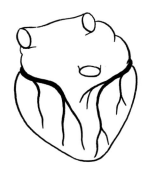

E ANT. INTERVENTRICULAR A.
FROM RIGHT CORONARY A.

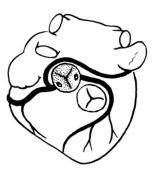

F LEFT CIRCUMFLEX CORONARY
ARTERY FROM RIGHT CORONARY A.

FIG. 73
Anomalies of the coronary arteries. (After Edwards et al., 1954, and Reemtsma et al., 1961.)

Rowlatt presents a careful description of the location of the aortic sinuses and the coronary arteries in transposition, and correlates the anomalies found with the internal anatomy present. The coronary pattern was particularly disturbed when the ventricular septum was abnormally formed; the pattern was unaffected by abnormality of the atrial septum or the atrioventricular orifices.

Several surgeons have attested to the danger, in operating for the tetralogy of Fallot, of accidentally dividing an anterior interventricular or the entire left coronary artery when these vessels take anomalous origin from the right coronary artery and then course to the left across the right ventricle (Kirklin *et al.,* 1959; Senning, 1959; Derrick *et al.,* 1963; Longenecker *et al.,* 1961; Reemtsma *et al.,* 1961). Senning also commented on one's incision being limited by such a vessel when it is recognized.

Examples of abnormal connection with the pulmonary artery or cardiac chambers are shown in Figure 74. Such communications are all said to be rare, the commonest being the origin of the left coronary from the pulmonary artery (Edwards, 1968). Origin of the right or of both coronary arteries from the pulmonary artery is extremely rare. These

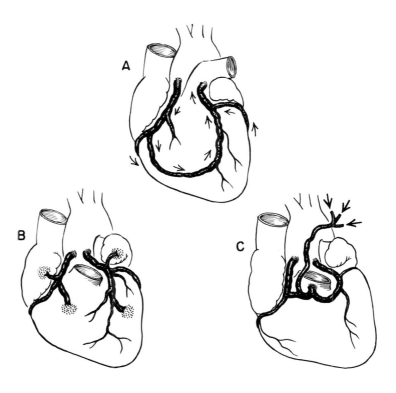

FIG. 74
Abnormal coronary artery communications. A. Left coronary artery originates in pulmonary artery. Arrows show direction of shunting. B. The coronary arteries communicate with the cardiac chambers. C. Both coronary arteries share a communication with the pulmonary artery. The arrows indicate additional shunting from pericardial vessels toward the pulmonary artery. (After Edwards et al., *1965.)*

connections constitute a distinct abnormality because differential pressure induces shunting from the coronary tree to the pulmonary artery or the right ventricle.

REFERENCES

Bland, E. F., White, P. D., and Garland, J.: Congenital anomalies of the coronary arteries. Report of an unusal case associated with cardiac hypertrophy. Amer. Heart J. 8:787–801, 1933.

Derrick, J. R., Cleveland, B. R., and Frazier, J.: Intramural and anomalous coronary arteries. Surgery 53:315–318, 1963.

Edwards, J. E.: Congenital Malformations of the Heart and Great Vessels. Chapter 9 *in* Pathology of the Heart, Gould, S. E., Ed., 3rd ed. Springfield, Charles C Thomas, 1968.

Edwards, J. E., Carey, L. S., Neufeld, H. N., and Lester, R. G.: Congenital Heart Disease. Correlation of Pathologic Anatomy and Angiocardiography. Vol. 2. Philadelphia, W. B. Saunders, 1965.

Edwards, J. E., Dry, T. J., Parker, R. L., Burchell, H. D., Wood, E. H., and Bulbulian, A. H.: An Atlas of Congenital Anomalies of the Heart and Great Vessels. Springfield, Charles C Thomas, 1954.

Geiringer, E.: The mural coronary. Amer. Heart J. 41:359–368, 1951.

Gerbode, F., Ross, J. K., March, H. W., Osborn, J. J., and Kerth, W. J.: Transverse ventriculotomy. Bull. Soc. Int. Chir. 21:345–353, 1962.

Kirklin, J. W., Ellis, F. H., Jr., McGoon, D. C., DuShane, J. W., and Swan, H. J. C.: Surgical treatment of the tetralogy of Fallot by open intracardiac repair. J. Thor. Surg. 37:22–51, 1959.

Krumbhaar, E. B., and Ehrich, W. E.: Varieties of single coronary artery in man, occurring as isolated cardiac anomalies. Am. J. Med. Sci. 196:407–413, 1938.

Longenecker, C. G., Reemtsma, K., and Creech, O., Jr.: Anomalous coronary artery distribution associated with tetralogy of Fallot: A hazard in open cardiac repair. J. Thorac. Cardiovasc. Surg. 42:258–262, 1961.

Meng, C. C. L., Eckner, F. A. O., and Lev, M.: Coronary artery distribution in tetralogy of Fallot. Arch. Surg. 90:363–366, 1965.

Reemtsma, K., Longenecker, C. G., and Creech, O., Jr.: Surgical anatomy of the coronary artery distribution in congenital heart disease. Circulation 24:782–787, 1961.

Roberts, J. T., and Loube, S. D.: Congenital single coronary artery in man. Report of nine new cases, one having thrombosis with right ventricular and atrial (auricular) infarction. Amer. Heart J. 34:188–208, 1947.

Rowlatt, U. F.: Coronary artery distribution in complete transposition. J.A.M.A. 179:269–278, 1962.

Senning, A.: Surgical treatment of right ventricular outflow tract stenosis combined with ventricular septal defect and right-left shunt (''Fallot's tetralogy''). Acta Chir. Scand. 117:73–81, 1959.

Trevor, R. S.: Congenital morbus cordis (cor biatriatum triloculare). Proc. Roy. Soc. Med. Vol. 5, Part 1, Section for Study of Disease in Children, pp. 26–28, 1912.

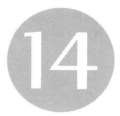

tHe cARdiAc coNduction system

LOCATION OF MAJOR COMPONENTS

The major tracts of specialized cardiac conduction tissues may be injured in the varied incisions and repairs undertaken in cardiac surgery. This is particularly important in operations for congenital heart disease. The pathologic studies of Lev (1962) clarify the location of the pathways in relation to congenital defects. Examples of inadvertent injury to the tracts have been published by Gerbode *et al.* (1962) and to their blood supply by Reemtsma *et al.* (1961). There are also uncommon indications for intentional surgical interruption of these pathways.

The specialized structures involved in cardiac conduction include the sinu-atrial node, the atrioventricular node, the atrioventricular bundle and its right and left branches, and the microscopic myofibril network of Purkinje (Fig. 75). Studies by James (1963a, b), Bowman and Malm (1965), and Holsinger *et al.* (1968) have confirmed the existence and surgical significance of the atrial internodal conduction tracts described by Keith and Flack (1907), Thorel (1909), and Wenckebach (1907). Additionally a tract has been described by Bachmann (1916) between the sinu-atrial node and the musculature of the left atrium (Fig. 75 A).

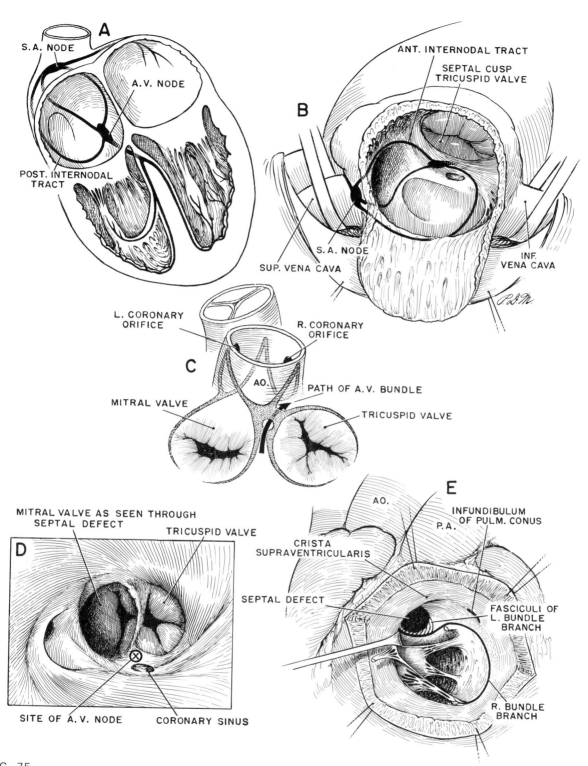

FIG. 75

The conduction system of the heart. A. A comprehensive diagrammatic view. B. The internodal pathways.
C. Path of the main atrioventricular bundle through the right fibrous skeletal trigone. D. Site of the atrioventricular
node in atrial septal defect of primum type. E. Relation of conduction elements to the interventricular septal defect
in tetralogy of Fallot.

The entire system is portrayed in Figure 75 A. The sinu-atrial node is a relatively large aggregation of cells extending laterally from the junction of the superior vena cava and the right atrial appendage to the sulcus terminalis and lying close to the epicardial surface. The possibility of injury to the node in passing a tape about the superior vena cava has been mentioned (p. 100; Fig. 59). Right atrial incisions should be designed to avoid the area of the node.

The node is connected to the surrounding atrial myo-cardium by ordinary muscle cells and to the atrioventricular node by three internodal pathways (Fig. 75 A and B), with some distribution to the adjacent muscle cells. The anterior tract curves forward from the sinu-atrial node along the upper margin of the interatrial septum at the base of the medial wall of the right atrial appendage, where it divides into a branch to the left atrium (Bachmann's bundle) and a branch that curves back into the anterior interatrial septum, behind the non-coronary cusp area of the aortic root, to enter the superior margin of the atrioventricular node. The middle tract curves behind the superior vena cava and thence courses anterior to the anulus fossae ovalis, to blend with fibers of the anterior tract as the atrioventricular node is approached. The posterior tract follows the crista terminalis inferiorly to the inferior caval (Eustachian) ridge, then courses along the ridge anterior to the coronary sinus to a point above the atrioventricular node, where it turns abruptly toward the node.

Free communication between the internodal tracts in the region of the atrioventricular node has been described by James (1961), who suggests that the node may be bypassed by some of these fibers during atrioventricular conduction. An incision in the right atrium that is extended through and across the interatrial septum for visualization of the mitral valve may divide all internodal tracts. Such instances, with atrioventricular dissociation, have been documented by Bowman and Malm (1965).

The atrioventricular node lies on the floor of the right atrium in the fibrous trigone between the ostium of the coronary sinus and the septal leaflet of the tricuspid valve (Fig. 75 B, C). The position of the node in a heart with an atrial defect of the septum primum type is shown in Figure 75 D. The bundle travels from this point along the right side of the ridge separating the mitral and tricuspid valves until it pierces the fibrous trigone. A patch for closure of a 'primum' defect should be placed on the left, or mitral, side.

The main atrioventricular bundle extends from the node to pierce the trigone (Fig. 75 C). Its length is frequently less than 1 cm. The bundle then enters the lower part of the membranous interventricular septum and is located beneath the junction of the right coronary and non-coronary aortic cusps where branching begins (Fig. 75 A). Injury to the atrioventricular bundle during prosthetic aortic valve replacement should be rare since the prosthesis is usually attached to the fibrous anulus, which is scalloped a centimeter or more above the bundle as it passes between the right coronary and non-coronary cusps. Severe calcification may distort this relationship. The suturing of a homograft aortic valve below the fibrous attachments of the aortic cusps is more hazardous to the main bundle.

Lev (1962) describes the initial branching of the common atrioventricular bundle into anterior and posterior radiations. The anterior radiation divides into fasciculi to the anterior papillary muscle of the left ventricle and the surrounding myocardium, then continues as the right bundle branch. The posterior radiation gives off fasciculi to the posterior papillary muscle and surrounding area of the left ventricle. There is a fanlike distribution of fasciculi from the left bundle as it passes along the inferior margin of the membranous interventricular septum (see Fig. 62). Its location in the tetralogy of Fallot is shown in Figure 75 E. Isolated left bundle branch block is not easily produced by sutures in this area because of the initial radiation. Complete block may occur when the atrioventricular node or common bundle is injured more proximally.

The right bundle branch is much more compact and passes just beneath the endocardium to the region of the conus papillary muscle where it moves deeper into the myocardium coursing along the lower border of the septal band of the crista supraventricularis to the moderator band. Interruption of the right bundle branch may occur fairly commonly with the repair of ventricular septal defect, but the resulting derangement is generally of little consequence. In the moderator band the right bundle branch again becomes subendocardial and divides into several branches.

Both the right and the left bundle branch terminate in a subendocardial network of Purkinje fibers.

INTENTIONAL INTERRUPTION OF CONDUCTION PATHWAYS

Bridges of conduction tissue between the right atrium and the lateral wall of the right ventricle have been described in a variety of mammalian species by Kent (1914). These bundles of ectopic conduction tissue have been found in some patients with ventricular pre-excitation (Wolff-Parkinson-White) syndrome. In a few instances surgical division of this tissue in the right atrioventricular groove has been performed for pre-excitation with tachycardia (Burchell *et al.,* 1967; Cobb *et al.,* 1968). Aberrant atrioventricular conduction might also result from functional bypass of the atrioventricular node, as suggested by James (1963a). Occasionally the surgical production of complete heart block by suture of the atrioventricular node or bundle may be necessary for the alleviation of life-threatening supraventricular tachycardia (Dreifus *et al.,* 1968).

REfERENCES

Bachmann, G.: The inter-auricular time interval. Am. J. Physiol. 41:309–320, 1916.

Bowman, F. O., Jr., and Malm, J.R.: The transseptal approach to mitral valve repair. Arch. Surg. 90:329–331, 1965.

Burchell, H. B., Frye, R. L., Anderson, M. W., and McGoon, D. C.: Atrioventricular and ventriculoatrial excitation in Wolff-Parkinson-White syndrome (type B). Temporary ablation at surgery. Circulation 36:663–672, 1967.

Cobb, F. R., Blumenschein, S. D., Sealy, W. C., Boineau, J. P., Wagner, G. S., and Wallace, A. G.: Successful surgical interruption of the bundle of Kent in a patient with Wolff-Parkinson-White syndrome. Circulation 38:1018–1029, 1968.

Dreifus, L. S., Nichols, H., Morse, D., Watanabe, Y., and Truex, R.: Control of recurrent tachycardia of Wolff-Parkinson-White syndrome by surgical ligature of the A-V bundle. Circulation 38:1030–1036, 1968.

Gerbode, F., Ross, J. K., March, H. W., Osborn, J. J., and Kerth, W. J.: Transverse ventriculotomy. Bull. Soc. Int. Chir. 21:345–353, 1962.

Holsinger, J. W., Jr., Wallace, A. G., and Sealy, W. C.: The identification and surgical significance of the atrial internodal conduction tracts. Ann. Surg. 167:447–453, 1968.

James, T. N.: Morphology of the human atrioventricular node, with remarks pertinent to its electrophysiology. Amer. Heart J. 62:756–771, 1961.

James, T. N.: The connecting pathways between the sinus node and A-V node and between the right and the left atrium in the human heart. Amer. Heart J. 66:498–508, 1963a.

James, T. N.: Anatomy of the conducting system of the heart. Heart Bull. 12:21–25, 1963b.

Keith, A., and Flack, M.: The form and nature of the muscular connections between the primary divisions of the vertebrate heart. J. Anat. Physiol. 41:172–189, 1907.

Kent, A. F. S.: The right lateral auriculo-ventricular junction of the heart. J. Physiol. 48:xxii–xxiv, 1914.

Lev, M.: The anatomy and pathology of the conduction system in the human heart. Hebrew Med. J. 1:243–262, 1962.

Reemtsma, K., Longenecker, C. G., and Creech, O., Jr.: Surgical anatomy of the coronary artery distribution in congenital heart disease. Circulation 24:782–787, 1961.

Thorel, C.: Vorläufige Mitteilung uber eine besondere Muskelverbindung zwischen der Cava superior und dem Hisschen Bündle. München. med. Wschr. 56:2159, 1909.

Wenckebach, K. F.: Beiträge zur Kenntnis der menschlichen Herztätigkeit. Arch. Anat. Physiol., Phys. Abt., pp. 1–24, 1907.

cardiac transplantation

The technique of cardiac transplantation shown (Fig. 76) is one suggested by Lower, Stofer, and Shumway (1961). Figure 76 A shows the cardiopulmonary bypass for the recipient and removal of the recipient's heart. The ascending aorta and the main pulmonary artery are divided. The atria are cut across at the atrioventricular sulcus, leaving intact the posterior walls of the atria and the interatrial septum.

In Figure 76 B the donor heart is removed with the entire right and left atria, short segments of the venae cavae, and longer portions of the ascending aorta and main pulmonary artery. This leaves intact the donor conduction mechanism and the coronary circulation. The donor atria are opened, avoiding the region of the sinu-atrial node. The interatrial septum is left intact, and the superior vena cava is ligated. Only four anastomoses are then required. The left atrial anastomosis is completed at the atrial septum of the recipient (Fig. 76 C). The right atrial anastomosis starts at this structure (Fig. 76 D).

For some weeks the remaining portions of the recipient's atria obtain their blood supply from mediastinal vessels which reach the atria on the walls of the pulmonary veins (see Fig. 58; pp. 98, 146).

Substantially the entire neural and lymphatic supply of the heart is interrupted at the arterial root, except for nerves and lymph vessels that may enter the remaining part of the

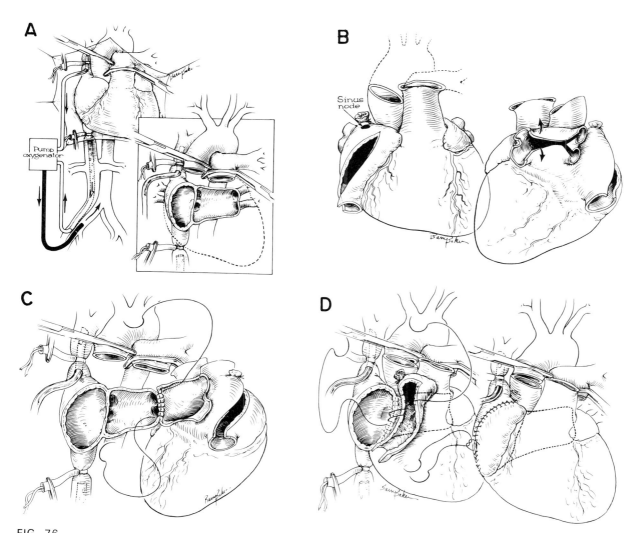

FIG. 76

Transplantation of the heart. A. The arrangement for cardiac bypass in the recipient. The insert shows portions of the atria and great vessels remaining after excision of the heart. B. The donor heart. The superior vena cava has been ligated, the right atrial incision extends through the cuff of the inferior cava. The left atrium has been opened widely into the cuffs of pulmonary veins. C. Beginning the anastomosis. Suturing of the left atria is begun at their left borders and completed at the atrial septum of the recipient. D. The anastomosis of the right atria begins at the atrial septum of the recipient. The aortae and pulmonary arteries await anastomosis. (From Cooley et al., 1969.)

left atrium from contiguous structures. According to Vasko (1969), the heart in animal experiments is re-innervated in months to years. Re-innervation of the transplanted human heart has not been demonstrated yet (Shaver *et al.,* 1969). Although the retained host atrial walls are rich in baro-receptors, it has not been shown that there remains any functionally significant transmission of their impulses. The interruption of cardiac lymphatics has been conjectured to be deleterious (Vasko, 1969).

REFERENCES

Cooley, D. A., Hallman, G. L., Bloodwell, R. D., Nora, J. J., and Leachman, R. D.: Cardiac transplantation as palliation of advanced heart disease. Arch. Surg. 98:619–625, 1969.

Lower, R. R., Stofer, R. C., and Shumway, N. E.: Homovital transplantation of the heart. J. Thorac. Cardiovasc. Surg. 41:196–204, 1961.

Shaver, J. A., Leon, D. F., Gray, S., III, Leonard, J. J., and Bahnson, H. T.: Hemodynamic observations after cardiac transplantation. New Eng. J. Med. 281:822–827, 1969.

Vasko, J. S.: Transplantation of the heart. Amer. J. Surg. 117:344–358, 1969.

16

THE CORONARY ARTERIES AND VEINS;
CARDIAC REVASCULARIZATION

PATTERNS OF CORONARY ARTERY
DISTRIBUTION

Whenever two or more vessels enter into collateral part-
nership there exists the possibility that one may be unusually
large or extensive in its distribution, with its partner being
proportionately diminutive (Fig. 77). Special vulnerability to
ischemia exists in the territory of meeting of the acral
branches of the partners, the 'junctional zone' (Edwards,
1958). For the heart the junctional zone is the interventricular septum. Piquand (1910) noted that one coronary artery
might be 'preponderant,' and supply more than the usual
part of the septum or adjacent ventricle. Schlesinger (1940)
emphasized that occlusion of a preponderant artery was more
likely to cause death than occlusion of a coronary artery in
a 'balanced' circulation, where the two arteries share the
supply to the septum in rather equal fashion—the left taking
care of the septum anteriorly, the right, posteriorly (Figs.
77–79). In 'right preponderance' the posterior interventricular artery derived from the right coronary artery supplies
much of the left ventricle as well (Fig. 77). In 'left preponderance' the posterior interventricular artery is a continuation of a large left circumflex branch (Figs. 77, 80). In such

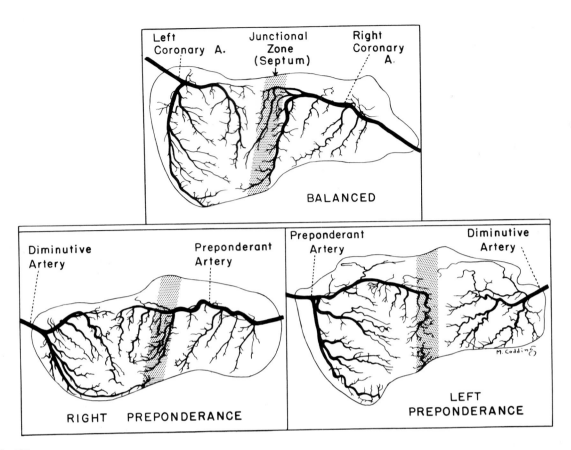

FIG. 77
Reciprocal relationship between the coronary arteries. (From Edwards, 1958; after Schlesinger, 1940.)

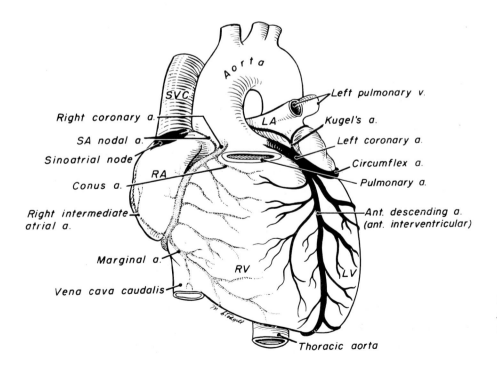

FIG. 78
Anterior view of coronary distribution of 'balanced' type. (From Truex, 1963.)

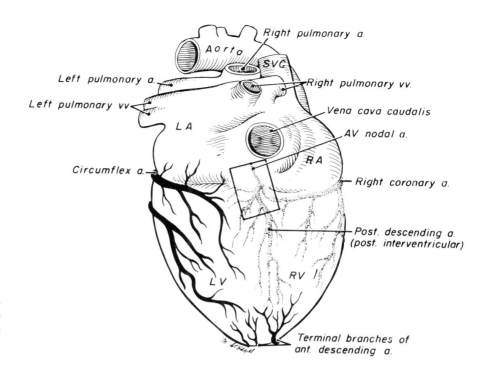

FIG. 79
Posterior view of coronary distribution of 'balanced' type. The 'crux' is indicated by the rectangle. (From Truex, 1963.)

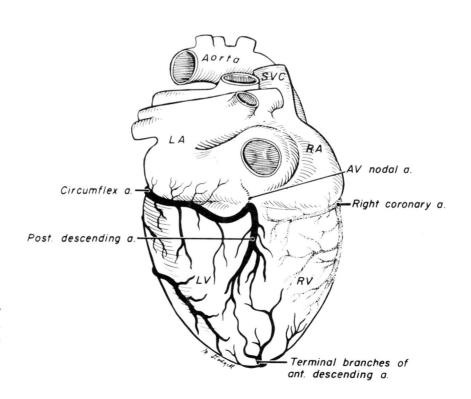

FIG. 80
Posterior view of a 'left preponderant' distribution. The artery of the atrioventricular node here derives from the left coronary artery. (From Truex, 1963.)

instances the artery of the atrioventricular node is derived from the left instead of the right coronary artery.

Schlesinger found that a 'balanced' circulation existed in 34 per cent of hearts, a 'right preponderance' in 48 per cent, and a 'left preponderance' in 18 per cent. Truex (1963) grants that the right preponderant coronary artery is of unusual significance, but states that even in these cases the greatest mass of heart muscle, which is left ventricular, still gets most of its supply from the left coronary artery.

BLOOD SUPPLY TO THE ATRIA AND NODAL TISSUE

Both coronary arteries give off branches to the atria. Two of these are noteworthy vessels: the sinu-atrial, the largest of the atrial branches, and the great auricular anastomotic (of Kugel), a smaller artery. The sinu-atrial artery arises in 60 per cent of cases from the proximal part of the right coronary artery. It supplies much of the aortic valve, right atrium, and the sinu-atrial node, and sends a branch across the anterior aspect of the left atrium to communicate with the left coronary artery. In the specimen pictured by Keith and Flack (1907), the connection between the two coronary arteries was so large as to constitute an origin for the sinu-atrial artery from each (Fig. 81). James and Burch (1958)

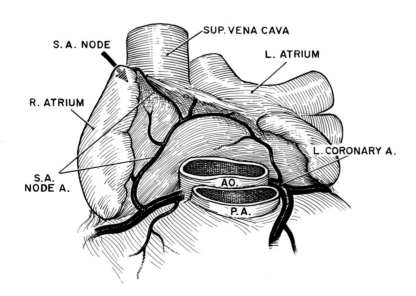

FIG. 81
Arteries to the sinu-atrial node. (After Keith and Flack, 1907.)

FIG. 82

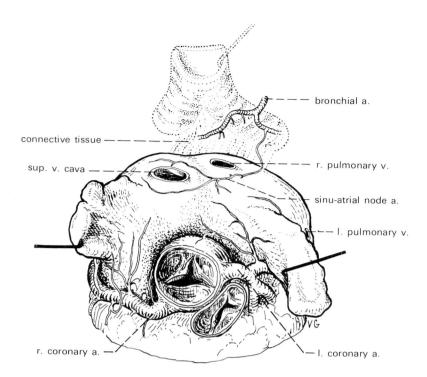

Figure labels: bronchial a., connective tissue, sup. v. cava, r. pulmonary v., sinu-atrial node a., l. pulmonary v., r. coronary a., VG, l. coronary a.

emphasize that procedures which impinge on the anterior interatrial groove may endanger the blood supply of the sinu-atrial node.

Details of coronary artery course and branching are beautifully shown by James (1961). The 'great auricular anastomotic artery' (Figs. 61, 78) was first described by Kugel (1928). It usually arises from the proximal portion of the left coronary artery, rarely from the right. It supplies some of the aortic valve, then courses in the interauricular area to reach the atrioventricular node, where it communicates with the artery to that node (see Fig. 61). It also communicates with the sinu-atrial node artery, and may be the source of that vessel.

An interesting example of origin of the sinu-atrial from a bronchial artery is shown in Figure 82. Such extracoronary vessels are further considered below.

Although earlier observations exist on the presence of a special artery to the atrioventricular node, the studies of James (1961) on this vessel are definitive. The artery is a branch of the right coronary in about 90 per cent. It arises from that vessel at the characteristic U-shaped bend of the posterior interventricular artery at the crux of the heart (junction of interatrial and interventricular septa and grooves) (see Fig. 79). It communicates with the great auricular anastomotic artery of Kugel (see Fig. 61). When there is 'preponderance' of the left coronary artery, the atrioventricular node artery arises from the left circumflex artery as it takes the U-shaped bend at the crux to furnish the posterior interventricular artery (Fig. 80).

Reemtsma *et al.* (1961) point out that the atrioventricular node artery may be injured in the closure of ostium primum defects, since it runs beneath the inferior rim of the defect.

NATURAL EXTERNAL COLLATERALS FOR THE CORONARY SYSTEM

Hudson *et al.* (1932) showed by postmortem injection that pericardial arteries reached the heart via the vasa vasorum of the major blood vessels passing through the pericardium (Fig. 58). Such communications constitute collaterals for the coronary system, and may provide the heart with a borderline circulation in those rare patients who survive occlusion of both coronary arteries. It would appear that such collaterals are the source of supply to the recipient atria after cardiac transplantation (Fig. 76).

Bjork (1966), by arteriography in living patients, showed communications between the coronary and extracoronary arteries (believed to be bronchial arteries) in over 25 per cent of patients with normal coronary vessels and in 50 per cent of those with coronary artery disease. In many of these latter patients the anastomoses were over 2 mm in diameter. Ovenfors (1956) also showed normal communications between the coronary sinus and mediastinal veins by coronary sinus phlebography.

The identity of the arteries involved is of considerable interest. Potential arteries supplying these communications include all branches from neighboring arteries to the pericardium. However, using postmortem angiography Moberg (1967a, b) found that the bronchial arteries supply the larger and most constant communications, those with the internal thoracic arteries being less constant. The bronchial arteries are more apt to communicate with atrial vessels, whereas the internal thoracic connect with both atrial and ventricular vessels. The communications of the bronchial and atrial vessels have a phylogenetic basis. In the rat, for example, the coronary arteries are regularly supplemented by an artery on each side stemming from the internal thoracic and dividing into bronchial and other mediastinal and atrial branches (Halpern, 1957).

Petelenz (1965a, b), by postmortem bronchial angiography in man, found that the bronchial arteries contributed substantially to the supply of the atria and especially of the sinu-atrial node. In 1909 Koch had found the sinu-atrial node artery totally derived from a bronchial artery in a human fetus. This was also true in Prof. Hromada's case (Fig. 82). Although he encountered this condition only once among 100 cases, he found the bronchial artery contributing substantially to the blood supply of the node in several others. These observations suggest that proximal division of the bronchial arteries might in some instances have a deleterious effect upon the node.

THE CORONARY VENOUS SINUS

The coronary sinus appears as a continuation of the great coronary vein (Fig. 83). On embryologic grounds its beginning is indicated by the termination of the oblique vein. The specimen drawn shows the small cardiac vein terminating in the middle cardiac, a fairly common pattern also shown by Adachi (1933). The anastomoses between coronary veins shown here is also usual. According to Adachi the diameter of the mid portion of the coronary sinus ranges from 7 to 14 mm (most often 8 to 10 mm); its length from the oblique vein to the entrance of the middle cardiac vein varies from 5 to 45 mm (most often from 15 to 30 mm).

Unicuspid or bicuspid valves are usually present at the mouths of the tributaries of the sinus. The great cardiac vein is most constantly thus equipped, contrary to the condition shown. The presence of a valve in the coronary sinus proper is most exceptional. Poirier *et al.* (1908) show a specimen like ours. There appears to be little evidence for the view frequently expressed that these venous valves are often incompetent. Their presence argues strongly against the occasional employment of retrograde perfusion of the coronary system through the sinus (Gott *et al.,* 1957). Such a practice

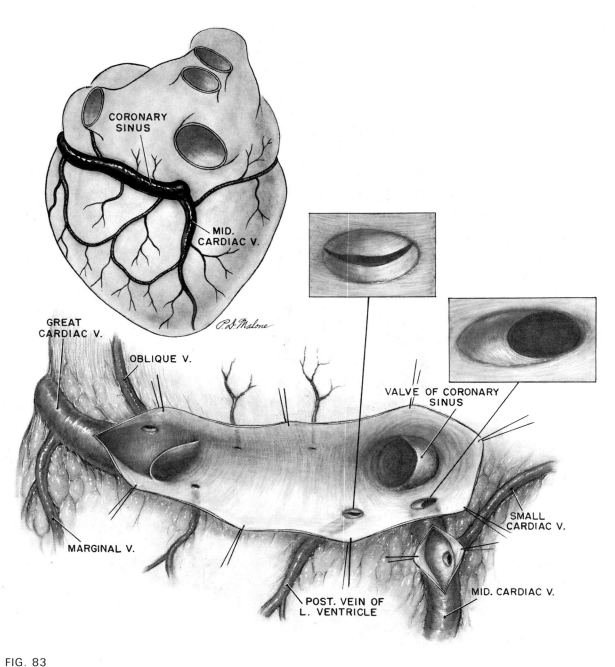

FIG. 83

The coronary venous system. The sinus is opened in the enlarged view below, to show the venous valves.

may produce incompetence of these venous valves. Fauteux in 1946 combined ligation of the great cardiac vein with pericoronary neurectomy for angina pectoris, a procedure that is not currently performed.

MYOCARDIAL REVASCULARIZATION

Operations to relieve myocardial ischemia include direct coronary artery reconstruction, and indirect techniques for anastomoses from extracoronary sources. Artery reconstruction is currently performed either by endarterectomy or by the placement of a graft (usually a segment of saphenous vein) between the ascending aorta and a coronary artery beyond the site of stenosis.

Each of the coronary arteries, the right and the left, measures 3 or 4 mm in internal diameter at birth, increasing with age. Diameters of about 1 cm recorded by Roessle and Roulet (1932) are probably abnormal. Two noteworthy observations on the venous relationships of the coronary arteries were made by Dr. Arlan Fuller in our laboratory. The proximal part of the anterior interventricular artery is often crossed superficially by the great cardiac vein. Any of the veins accompanying the major arteries may be doubled. The middle cardiac vein is particularly likely to possess this pattern; thus two veins may accompany the posterior interventricular artery.

Claude Beck has performed an extraordinary number of studies in the production of communications between extracoronary arteries and the coronary system. Pedicles of pectoral muscle, omentum, spleen, lung (in the hope of bronchial artery connections) have been employed; and adhesions between parietal and visceral pericardium have been encouraged, to foster vascular connections through the pericardial vessels. For a time the internal thoracic arteries were ligated distal to the origin of the pericardiacophrenic arteries in the hope of increasing flow to the pericardium, and thus to the heart, via the vasa vasorum at the pericardial reflections (see Fig. 58).

At present, the most widely performed operation based on a pedicled source of extracoronary blood flow is the implantation of one or both internal thoracic arteries into a myocardial tunnel ('the Vineberg procedure') (Vineberg,

1964). The intramural or other anomalous course of the coronary arteries (see Fig. 72) must be kept in mind. In the procedure the cut ends of the branches of the internal thoracic artery are left open to perfuse the sinusoids of the myocardium (Fig. 84). The sinusoids in turn connect with both coronary arterioles and veins (Wearn *et al.,* 1933). Generally, a pedicle is fashioned of the internal thoracic artery and its venae comitantes and adjacent fat. Sewell (1967) leaves longer segments of the intercostal vessels attached to the internal thoracic artery to produce his 'triple pedicle.' The internal thoracic artery may be left attached to the chest wall below rather than above, to receive supply from its superior epigastric and musculophrenic

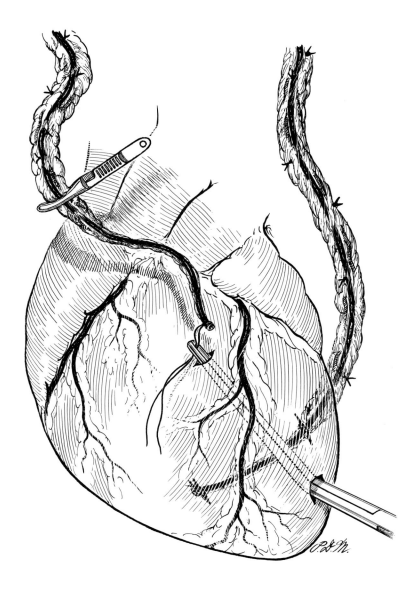

FIG. 84
Myocardial revascularization by intramural placement of the internal thoracic (internal mammary) vessels ('Vineberg procedure'). The terminal ligature will remain. The orifices of branches of the implanted artery are left open.

branches, but pressure and flow are probably less in this case. The approach is usually mid sternal (see Fig. 56), with the internal thoracic vessels dissected from the underside of each sternocostal mass. The lower segments of these vessels are disclosed by incising the sternocostal or transversus thoracis muscle which covers them.

REFERENCES

Adachi, B.: Das Venensystem der Japaner. Tokyo, Kenkyusha, 1933.

Björk, L.: Angiographic demonstration of extracardial anastomoses to the coronary arteries. Radiology 87:274–277, 1966.

Edwards, E. A.: The anatomy of collateral circulation. Surg. Gynec. Obstet. 107:183–194, 1958.

Fauteux, M.: Surgical treatment of angina pectoris. Experiences with ligation of the great cardiac vein and pericoronary neurectomy. Ann. Surg. 124:1041–1046, 1946.

Gott, V. L., Gonzales, J. L., Zuhdi, M. N., Varco, R. L., and Lillehei, C. W.: Retrograde perfusion of the coronary sinus for direct vision aortic surgery. Surg. Gynec. Obstet. 104:319–328, 1957.

Halpern, M. H.: The dual blood supply of the rat heart. Amer. J. Anat. 101:1–16, 1957.

Hudson, C. L., Moritz, A. R., and Wearn, J. T.: The extracardiac anastomoses of the coronary arteries. J. Exp. Med. 56:919–925, 1932.

James, T. N.: Anatomy of the Coronary Arteries. New York, Hoeber, 1961.

James, T. N., and Burch, G. E.: The atrial coronary arteries in man. Circulation 17:90–98, 1958.

Keith, A., and Flack, M.: The form and nature of the muscular connections between the primary divisions of the vertebrate heart. J. Anat. Physiol. 41:172–189, 1907.

Koch, W.: Ueber die Blutversorgung des Sinusknotens und etwaige Beziehungen des letzteren zum Atrioventrikularknoten. München. med. Wschr. 56:2362–2364, 1909.

Kugel, M. A.: Anatomical studies on the coronary arteries and their branches. I. Arteria anastomotica auricularis magna. Amer. Heart J. 3:260–270, 1928.

Moberg, A.: Anastomoses between extracardiac vessels and coronary arteries. I. Via bronchial arteries. Acta Radiol. Diagn. 6:177–192, 1967a.

Moberg, A.: Anastomoses between extracardiac vessels and coronary arteries. II. Via internal mammary arteries. Post-mortem angiographic study. Acta Radiol. Diagn. 6:263–272, 1967b.

Ovenfors, C.-O.: Venous communications between the cardiac veins and the large venous trunks in the superior part of the mediastinum. Acta Radiol. 46:518–522, 1956.

Petelenz, T.: Radiological picture of extracoronary arteries of myocardium in man. Cardiologia 46:65–78, 1965a.

Petelenz, T.: Extracoronary blood supply of the sinu-atrial (Keith-Flack's) node. Cardiologia 47:57–67, 1965b.

Piquand, G.: Recherches sur l'anatomie des vaisseaux sanguins du coeur. J. Anat. Phys. 46:310–340, 1910.

Poirier, P., Charpy, A., and Cunéo, B.: Abrégé d'anatomie. Vol. 2. Paris, Masson & Cie, 1908.

Reemtsma, K., Longenecker, C. G., and Creech, O., Jr.: Surgical anatomy of the coronary artery distribution in congenital heart disease. Circulation 24:782–787, 1961.

Roessle, R., and Roulet, F.: Mass und Zahl in der Pathologie. Berlin, Springer, 1932.

Schlesinger, M. J.: Relation of anatomic pattern to pathologic conditions of the coronary arteries. Arch. Path. 30:403–415, 1940.

Sewell, W. H.: Surgery for Acquired Coronary Disease. Springfield, Charles C Thomas, 1967.

Truex, R. C.: The Distribution of the Human Coronary Arteries. Pp. 4–10 in Coronary Heart Disease, Likoff, W., and Moyer, J. H., Eds. New York, Grune & Stratton, 1963.

Vineberg, A.: Experimental background of myocardial revascularization by internal mammary artery implantation and supplementary technics, with its clinical application in 125 patients. A review and critical appraisal. Ann. Surg. 159:185–207, 1964.

Wearn, J. T., Mettier, S. R., Klumpp, T. G., and Zschiesche, L. J.: The nature of the vascular communications between the coronary arteries and the chambers of the heart. Amer. Heart J. 9:143–164, 1933.

cARdiAC iNNERVATION

The sources of the innervation of the heart are the upper four (some say five) intercostal nerves of both sides for pain sensation and sympathetic innervation, and the vagus nerves for pressure sensory reception and parasympathetic control (Fig. 85). Cardiac branches from these sources reach the cardiac plexus (Fig. 86) about the pulmonary arteries and arch of the aorta to be distributed via the two coronary plexuses.

Mizeres (1963) called attention to the fact that the cardiac plexus is mainly located about the main pulmonary artery and its bifurcation, where it is actually combined with the pulmonary plexuses on each side. This is the part formerly named deep cardiac plexus and described as lying on the bifurcation of the trachea. Several cardiac nerves do lie in front of the trachea on their way to the plexus. A smaller part of the plexus, formerly called superficial cardiac plexus, lies antero-inferior to the arch of the aorta, and joins the main part below. An inconstant 'cardiac ganglion' (of Wrisberg) may lie in the plexus below the aortic arch.

The sympathetic fibers pass through the upper four intercostal nerves to reach the three cervical sympathetic ganglia (Fig. 85). Each ganglion gives off a cardiac branch (the superior, middle, and inferior, respectively). These descend behind the carotid arteries or within the carotid sheath, combining variously with cardiac branches of the vagus before

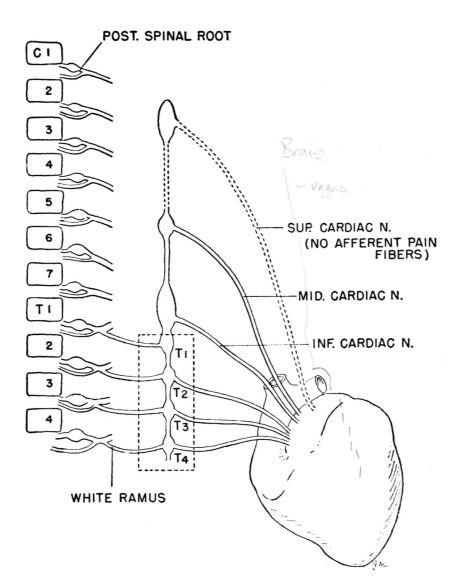

POST. SPINAL ROOT

C1
2
3
4
5
6
7
T1
2
3
4

WHITE RAMUS

Brain

Vagus

SUP. CARDIAC N.
(NO AFFERENT PAIN
FIBERS)

MID. CARDIAC N.

INF. CARDIAC N.

T1
T2
T3
T4

FIG. 85
Cardiac branches from the cervical and thoracic sympathetic trunk. (From Evans et al., 1950.) The direct extrapleural branches from the upper thoracic sympathetic chain are not shown. The sympathetic cardiac nerves carry both sensory and sympathetic (motor) fibers. The dotted rectangle indicates the extent of neurectomy recommended for the relief of angina.

reaching the cardiac plexus. Multiple delicate cardiac branches also leave the upper thoracic segments of the sympathetic trunk to course directly under the pleura to reach the hilar structures of the lung and the aorta, and thus contribute to the cardiac plexus. The pain fibers arise from the posterior root ganglia of the upper four or five intercostal nerves and utilize the conduits of the sympathetic system to reach the heart. They thus go through the white rami communicantes to the sympathetic chain and are distributed through all the sympathetic cardiac nerves mentioned above, except the superior cervical cardiac nerves, which are said not to carry pain fibers.

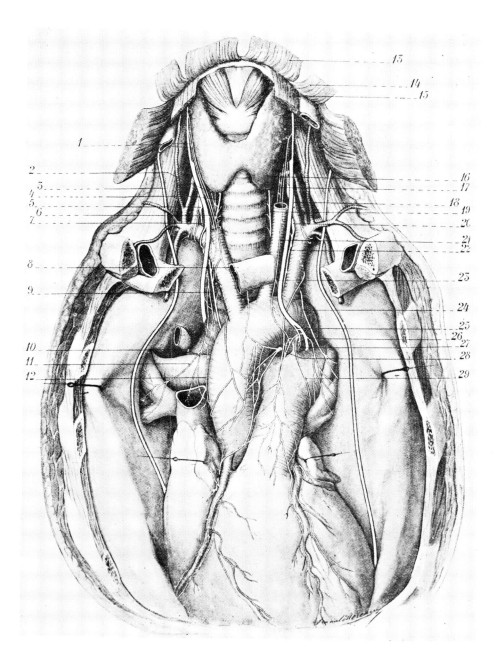

FIG. 86

The cardiac plexus.   1, superior vagal cardiac nerves; 2, middle sympathetic cardiac nerve; 3, phrenic nerve; 4, middle sympathetic cardiac nerve; 5, middle cervical ganglion; 6, recurrent laryngeal nerve; 7, inferior sympathetic cardiac nerve; 8, left brachiocephalic vein; 9, common trunk formed by the three sympathetic cardiac nerves; 10, 11, 12, branches of the inferior vagal cardiac nerves to the superior vena cava, lung, right bronchus, and pulmonary artery; 13, 14, 15, sternohyoid, omohyoid, and sternothyroid muscles; 16, 17, superior and middle sympathetic cardiac nerves; 18, middle cervical ganglion; 19, recurrent laryngeal nerve; 20, stellate ganglion; 21, superior vagal cardiac nerve; 22, inferior sympathetic cardiac nerve; 23, anastomosis between the superior vagal, and the superior and middle sympathetic cardiac nerves; 24, pulmonary branches of the inferior sympathetic cardiac nerve; 25, anastomosis between the vagus and the recurrent laryngeal nerve; 26, common trunks formed by the left inferior cardiac nerves and pulmonary branches; 27, middle vagal cardiac nerves; 28, the 'cardiac ganglion' (of Wrisberg); 29, vagal branches to the left bronchus and left pulmonary artery. (From Hovelacque, 1927.)

The cardiac efferent (parasympathetic) fibers of the vagus course in the vagal cardiac nerves, which are of variable number. They are given off, both high and low in the neck, from the recurrent laryngeal nerve of each side, and from the vagus trunks in the thorax. These latter two groups, on the left side, may be termed thoracic cardiac branches, and the term is also applied to other branches of the thoracic portion of the vagus, especially offshoots of the pulmonary plexuses. The sensory fibers of the vagus are those carrying stretch and pressure information. The cell bodies for these fibers lie in the vagal ganglia in the upper part of the cervical course of these nerves. Knowledge of the location of the receptor areas comes mainly from animal experimentation. Nonidez (1937a, b) indicated that the areas are located in the arch of the aorta, the site of origin of the right subclavian artery, the ligamentum arteriosum, the posterior parts of both atria with their entering veins, and the sinu-atrial node.

Mizeres detailed some of the combinations of the vagal and sympathetic branches prior to their reaching the cardiac plexus. Most of the cardiac nerves of the left side pass behind the arch of the aorta; those of the right side may lie somewhat to the right behind the brachiocephalic or the right subclavian artery. Some cardiac nerves may course anterior to the subclavian arteries with the vagus nerves. The plexus on the arch of the aorta carries more fibers from the left vagus and sympathetic trunk than from those on the right.

The distribution to the heart of nerves from the cardiac plexus is mainly through the subsidiary right and left coronary plexuses. Mizeres states that a few filaments go directly to the right and left atria, some coursing through the oblique ligament (of Marshall) of the left atrium. Physiological evidence (Wiggers, 1949) indicates that the sinu-atrial node is supplied mainly from the right vagus and the right sympathetic trunk, while the atrioventricular node and bundles are supplied from the vagus and sympathetic trunk of the left side.

Cardiac pain is effectively relieved by bilateral cervicodorsal sympathectomy removing the stellate and the second, third, and fourth ganglia (White *et al.*, 1933). Evans and Poppen (1953) note that the removal of the stellate ganglion alone, first done by Jonnesco in 1920, often failed to relieve pain. Denervation may be inadequate if one does not remove the fourth thoracic ganglion. The bilaterality of sensory innervation is considered by Wyburn-Mason (1950). He found that anginal pain was felt on the left or right, depending on the side of the heart suffering the severest ischemia. He cites an interesting case of right-sided pain in a patient with dextrocardia where the ischemic major ventricle was right sided. A cervicodorsal sympathectomy to relieve pain can be done by either the scalene approach, a high lateral thoracotomy, or an extrapleural thoracotomy (pp. 16 *et seq.*).

Fauteux and Swenson (1946) attempted to relieve anginal pain by pericoronary neurectomy. This approach has not been exploited by others. It is reasonable to presume that some denervation, sensory or motor, may accompany any periarterial dissection along the arch of the aorta, or along the pulmonary or coronary arteries. Cardiac transplantation represents a massive interruption of all known nerve pathways. It is probable that the posterior portions of the host atria, left intact in the Shumway technique (see Fig. 76), are minimally innervated from the adjacent cardiac and pulmonary plexuses.

REfERENCES

Evans, J. A., and Poppen, J. L.: Resection of anginal pathway for relief of anginal pain. New Eng. J. Med. 249:791–796, 1953.

Evans, J. A., Poppen, J. L., and Tobias, J. B.: Relief of angina pectoris by sympathectomy. Report of results in ten patients subjected to high thoracolumbar sympathectomy including the anginal pathway. J.A.M.A. 144:1432–1436, 1950.

Fauteux, M., and Swenson, O.: Pericoronary neurectomy in abolishing anginal pain in coronary disease. An experimental evaluation. Arch. Surg. 53:169–181, 1946.

Hollinshead, W. H.: Textbook of Anatomy, 2nd ed. New York, Harper & Row, Hoeber Medical Division, 1967.

Hovelacque, A.: Anatomie des nerfs craniens et rachidiens et du système grand sympathique. Paris, Doin, 1927.

Mizeres, N. J.: The cardiac plexus in man. Amer. J. Anat. 112:141–151, 1963.

Nonidez, J. F.: Distribution of the aortic nerve fibers and the epithelioid bodies (supracardial 'paraganglia') in the dog. Anat. Rec. 69:299–315, 1937a.

Nonidez, J. F.: Identification of the receptor areas in the venae cavae and pulmonary veins which initiate reflex cardiac acceleration (Bainbridge's reflex). Amer. J. Anat. 61:203–231, 1937b.

White, J. C., Garrey, W. E., and Atkins, J. A.: Cardiac innervation. Experimental and clinical studies. Arch. Surg. 26:765–786, 1933.

Wiggers, C. J.: Physiology in Health and Disease, 5th ed. Philadelphia, Lea & Febiger, 1949.

Wyburn-Mason, R.: Significance of the reference of anginal pain to the right or left side of the body. Amer. Heart J. 39:325–335, 1950.

18

lymphatics of the heart

The lymphatic vessels draining the heart lie in the sub-epicardial tissue and combine to form two collecting trunks: an anterior in the right coronary groove, and a posterior in the left (Fig. 87). As these trunks are developed an intercalated lymph node may occasionally be present.

The anterior trunk drains mainly the territory of the right coronary artery. The trunk ascends on the anterior surface of the ascending aorta, and then on its arch behind the thymus and the anterior edges of the pleurae, to terminate in the middle of a group of nodes lying below and parallel to the left brachiocephalic vein. These nodes are termed anterior mediastinal, and are to be distinguished from the parasternal nodes.

The posterior trunk drains the territory of the left coronary artery. It ascends on the posterior aspect of the main pulmonary artery deep to the pericardium forming the roof of the transverse sinus, and then on the right pulmonary artery beyond the pericardium. Rouvière (1932) stated that the posterior trunk ends in a node below and to the left of the tracheal bifurcation (Fig. 87). Shore (1929) found it terminating more frequently in the 'caval cardiac node,' the lowest member of the right superior tracheobronchial group. It lies above the right bronchus and pulmonary artery, behind the superior vena cava and adjacent aorta.

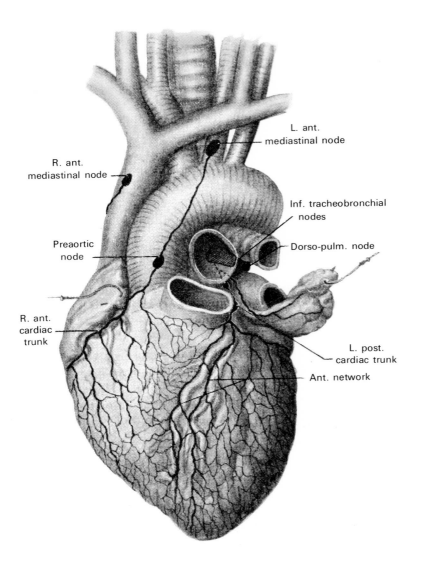

R. ant.
mediastinal node —

L. ant.
— mediastinal node

Inf. tracheobronchial
nodes

Preaortic
node

Dorso-pulm. node

R. ant.
cardiac
trunk

L. post.
cardiac trunk

Ant. network

FIG. 87
Lymphatics of the heart. (*From Rouvière, 1932.*)

Experimental work in the dog (Miller *et al.,* 1961; Symbas *et al.,* 1969) indicates that lymphatic obstruction may cause significant endocardial fibrosis, and disturbed atrioventricular valve function.

The anterior collecting trunk may be disturbed in exposures of the aorta, the posterior, in mobilizing the pulmonary artery. Both trunks are of course divided and then oversewn at the arterial anastomoses of the transplanted heart.

References

Miller, A. J., Pick, R., and Katz, L. N.: Lymphatics of the mitral valve of the dog. Demonstration and discussion of the possible significance. Circ. Res. 9:1005–1009, 1961.

Rouvière, H.: Anatomie des lymphatiques de l'homme. Paris, Masson, 1932.

Shore, L. R.: The lymphatic drainage of the human heart. J. Anat. 63:291–313, 1929.

Symbas, P. N., Schlant, R. C., Gravanis, M. B., and Shepherd, R. L.: Pathologic and functional effects on the heart following interruption of the cardiac lymph drainage. J. Thorac. Cardiovasc. Surg. 57:577–584, 1969.

pericardiocentesis
and drainage

APPROACHES

The subxiphoid route is the safest for pericardiocentesis (Fig. 88 C). The patient should be recumbent, with the thorax and head elevated 15 to 20 degrees from the horizontal. In this position fluid in the pericardium tends to accumulate just above the diaphragm. The needle is introduced in the space between the xiphoid process and the left seventh costal cartilage. It is advanced at approximately 30 degrees elevation from the skin surface and directed about 30 degrees to the left of the longitudinal axis.

The needle traverses the subcutaneous tissue and rectus sheath and muscle, and passes above the diaphragm to the fibrous pericardium. Hugging the posterior surface of the cartilage avoids the peritoneum (Fig. 88 C, D). A change in resistance is felt when the pericardium is punctured. The point of the needle is now advanced toward the junction of the anterior and diaphragmatic surfaces of the ventricle, an area in which no major coronary vessel should be encountered.

Compare this with the often-recommended parasternal puncture shown in Figure 88 A. As shown in Figures 56, 57 the interpleural space is variable, making the occurrence of pneumothorax a distinct possibility. Additionally, the anterior

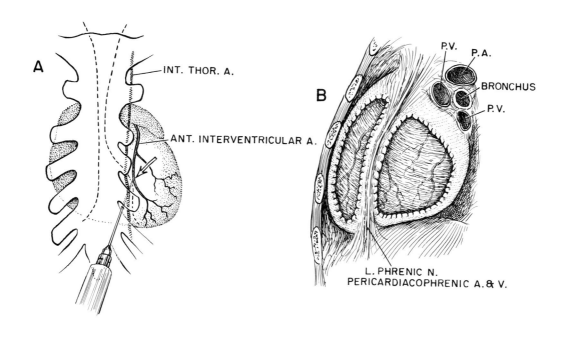

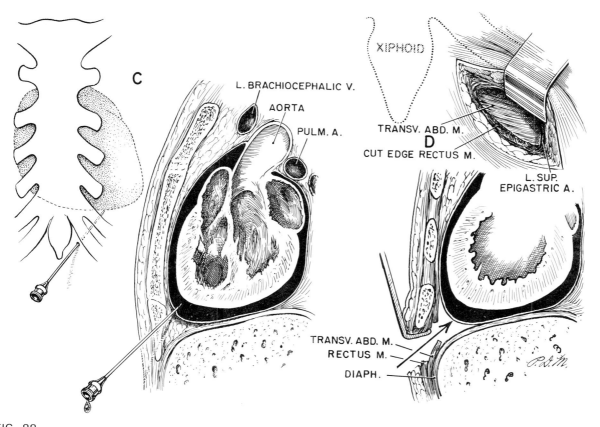

FIG. 88

Pericardial puncture, drainage, and excision. A. Demonstrates the dangers of a parasternal puncture. B. Peri-cardiectomy for effusion. C. Subxiphoid pericardiocentesis. D. Subxiphoid drainage.

interventricular vessels lie directly in the needle's path. In the specimen drawn, the needle point perforated the anterior interventricular artery. The internal thoracic vessels are avoided in this technique, if the puncture is made close to the sternum.

Open drainage of the pericardium may be accomplished by providing a communication to the pleural space. Alternately it may be drained without entering the pleural space by a left subcostal approach (Fig. 88 D). This is the same path used for subxiphoid puncture. After the fibers of the rectus abdominis and transversus muscles have been divided, the epiphrenic fat is dissected to expose the parietal pericardium, which may then be incised.

PERICARDIECTOMY FOR EFFUSION

Pericardiectomy for effusion is shown in Figure 88 B. Large windows have been removed anterior and posterior to the pericardiacophrenic neurovascular bundle. A bridge of pericardium is left beneath the bundle to protect these structures from stretching during surgery. The cut edges of pericardium are oversewn to ensure hemostasis. Such extensive fenestration over the left ventricle gives protection against later pericardial constriction of this chamber. If herniation of the heart should occur, the pericardium may become a tight band around the atrioventricular groove, interfering severely with cardiac output. The chance of herniation is reduced by preserving the phrenic bridge and supporting the apex in the sling of pericardium.

Pericardiectomy for constrictive pericarditis should include more extensive resection than the operation for effusion shown in Figure 88 B. The left ventricle and atrioventricular groove bilaterally must be liberated. In some instances, also, scarred bands restricting flow through the superior or inferior vena cava or compressing the right ventricular outflow tract need excision. Because of the more complete access available, median sternotomy is, in most instances, the best approach for constrictive pericarditis.

SECTION 4

Lungs and Trachea

pulmonary lobes and segments; bronchoscopy

LOBES AND FISSURES

There is great similarity in the lobar configuration of the bronchovascular distribution to the two lungs. The lingular portion of the left upper lobe corresponds to the middle lobe of the right lung. Rarely the lingula may exist as a separate lobe, demarcated by a horizontal fissure.

The oblique fissure (Fig. 89) separates the lower lobe from the upper and middle lobes of the right and from the upper lobe of the left lung. On the right side, the oblique fissure extends from the fourth thoracic vertebral spine posteriorly to the costochondral junction of the sixth rib. The horizontal fissure runs from the sixth rib in the mid-axillary line to the fourth costochondral junction anteriorly. The left oblique fissure lies more vertically than the right. It may start higher and ends on the costal arch at the seventh costal cartilage.

The fissures vary in depth. The right horizontal fissure is often incomplete, but a connective tissue plane may indicate the demarcation of the lobes. When a fissure is incomplete, an interlobar vein may be present. The right horizontal fissure may be occupied deeply by an anterior segmental vein of the upper lobe.

Accessory lobes may be present. An azygos lobe (Fig.

90) occurs in about 0.5 per cent of persons. The lobe is formed by indentation of the right upper lobe by the arch of the azygos vein lying in a fold of parietal pleura, the mesoazygos. Except for the azygos, most accessory lobes, such as the lingular or a basal cardiac lobe, represent demarcation of segments from the parent lobe (Hollinshead, 1956).

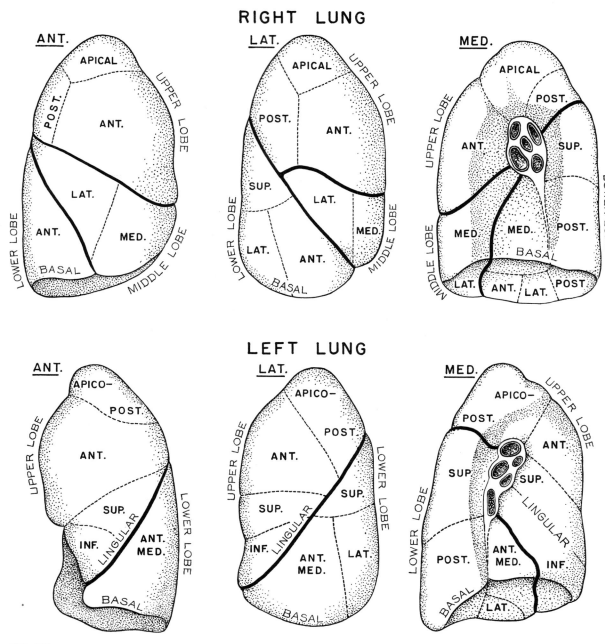

FIG. 89
Pulmonary lobes and segments. (After Wareham and Huse, 1964.)

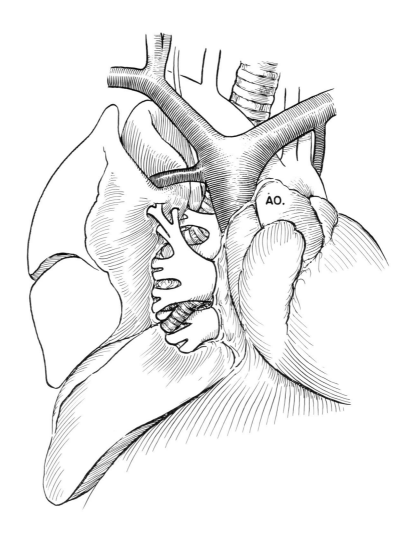

FIG. 90
Azygos lobe. (After Adachi, 1933.)

SEGMENTS

The lung segment represents to the surgeon a portion of a lobe sufficiently delimited in its bronchovascular supply to allow its resection without significant injury to the remaining adjacent portions. The pattern of bronchus and vessels is repetitive for each segment, smaller divisions termed subsegments, and for the lobules. For the lobules, the division of the bronchial tree becomes a bronchiole devoid of cartilage. In each of these divisions of the lobe, the artery and bronchus are arranged in a central 'ray,' and the vein is located between segments or lobules. The circumscription of lung tissue is best realized for the bronchus. This is shown by collapse of the segment when its bronchus is occluded at operation, the rest of the lobe being expanded by intratracheal insufflation (see Fig. 109). Exceptionally, air from adjacent segments may enter a segment through anomalous small bronchi, or through interalveolar openings, the 'alveolar pores' (of Kohn).

The segmental artery is quite well circumscribed in its distribution, but some communication with arteries of adjacent segments may exist.

Peripherally, the veins are intersegmental, receiving tributaries from adjacent segments. Subpleural tributaries are small, becoming prominent only as a result of local pathologic change. Naming a vein for a particular segment indicates only the preponderance of that segment over another in its field of drainage.

The segments and their bronchi and blood vessels are subject to considerable variation, leading to some differences in nomenclature. The Jackson-Huber (1943) system generally used in the United States recognizes 10 segments on the right and 8 on the left. These are shown in Figure 89 and tabulated in Figure 91 A. Note that for the apex of the lungs there are an apical and a posterior segment on the right and a single apicoposterior segment on the left, although left apical and posterior subsegments remain, with variable bronchial supply. In the lower lobes, the anterior and medial basal segments of the right lung correspond to the single anterior-medial basal segment of the left.

Variations have been carefully studied and documented by Boyden (1955). The text by Bloomer and his associates (1960) is also helpful.

BRONCHOSCOPY

The appearance of the orifices of the segmental bronchi as seen through the bronchoscope is shown in Figure 91 B. With the subject in the upright position, the tracheal bifurcation lies at the level of the sixth or seventh thoracic vertebra, but in the supine position it rises to the fourth vertebra. As the bronchoscope is passed through the tracheal lumen the median ridge, called the carina, is encountered. Turning the head to the right or left inclines the instrument for passage down the left or right principal bronchus, respectively. The upper lobe bronchi are visualized by using a telescope with an

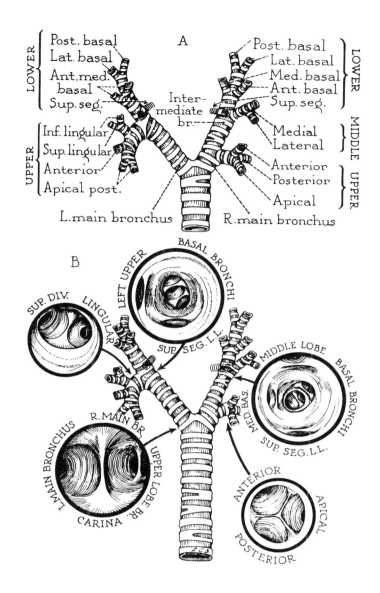

FIG. 91
Lobar and segmental bronchi, identified by name (A), and showing bronchoscopic views at various levels (B). (From Wareham and Huse, 1964.)

angled viewing lens. The right principal bronchus is wider, shorter, and more nearly vertical than the left. This accounts for the higher incidence of aspiration of foreign material into the right lung and the more common occurrence of abscesses on the right side. About 2 cm from its origin, the right principal bronchus gives rise to the upper lobe bronchus, which quickly divides into branches to the apical, anterior, and posterior segments. The right upper lobe bronchus was called the eparterial bronchus by Aeby (1880) because the pulmonary artery passes in a groove across the anterior surface of the intermediate bronchus below its origin (see Fig. 92). The bronchi to the middle lobe and superior segment of the lower lobe arise at nearly the same level, proceeding anterolaterally and posteromedially, respectively. The lower lobe bronchus then gives origin to the basal segmental bronchi, as illustrated.

The left principal bronchus pursues a less vertical course for 4 to 6 cm before the upper lobe bronchus originates. Enlargement of the left atrium may push the principal bronchus further upward, until it is nearly horizontal. The superior division of the left upper lobe bronchus gives rise to the anterior and apicoposterior segmental bronchi. The inferior division branches into the superior and inferior lingular bronchi. Less than 1 cm distal to the left upper lobe orifice, the superior segmental bronchus of the lower lobe arises. The lower lobe bronchus then terminates by giving rise to the basal bronchi.

REFERENCES

Adachi, B.: Das Venensystem der Japaner. Tokyo, Kenkyusha, 1933.

Aeby, C.: Der Bronchialbaum der Säugethiere und des Menschen, nebst Bemerkungen über der Vögel und Reptilien. Leipzig, Engelmann, 1880.

Bloomer, W. E., Liebow, A. A., and Hales, M. R.: Surgical Anatomy of the Bronchovascular Segments. Springfield, Charles C Thomas, 1960.

Boyden, E. A.: Segmental Anatomy of the Lungs. A Study of the Patterns of the Segmental Bronchi and Related Pulmonary Vessels. New York, McGraw-Hill Book Co., Blakiston Division, 1955.

Hollinshead, W. H.: Anatomy for Surgeons. Vol. 2, The Thorax, Abdomen, and Pelvis. New York, Hoeber, 1956.

Jackson, C. L., and Huber, J. F.: Correlated applied anatomy of the bronchial tree and lungs with a system of nomenclature. Dis. Chest 9:319–326, 1943.

Wareham, E. E., and Huse, W. M.: Surgical anatomy of the lungs. Surg. Clin. N. Amer. 44:1191–1200, 1964.

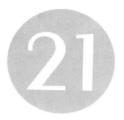

THE LUNG pEdiCLE ANd PULMONARY RESECTIONS

The pedicle of the lung may be considered as one single structure—the 'root' of the lung—as it emerges from the mediastinum, or as a group of constituent structures in the hilum as the bronchus and vessels give off lobar and segmental branches. The first viewpoint is particularly useful in planning total pneumonectomy—the second, in considering lobectomy or segmental resection.

THE ROOT OF THE LUNG

As it extends from lung to mediastinum, the root of the lung is surrounded by the pleura. The inferior aspect of the reflected pleura is redundant and is called the pulmonary ligament. Figure 92 shows the right lung root lying below the arch of the azygos vein; behind the superior vena cava, both atria, and more distantly the phrenic nerve; and in front of the vertical portions of the azygos, the esophagus, and the right vagus nerve. The root of the left lung (Fig. 93) lies below the arch of the aorta, to which it is attached by the ligamentum arteriosum, and is here related to the branching of the recurrent laryngeal nerve from the left vagus. It lies behind the left atrium and main pulmonary

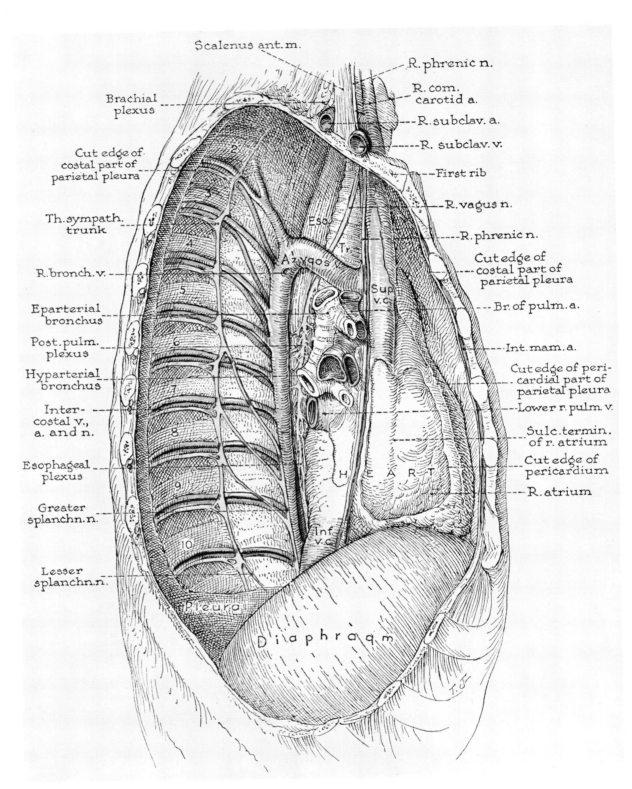

Scalenus ant. m.

R. phrenic n.

Brachial
plexus

R. com.
carotid a.

R. subclav. a.

R. subclav. v.

Cut edge of
costal part of
parietal pleura

First rib

R. vagus n.

Th. sympath.
trunk

R. phrenic n.

Cut edge of
costal part of
parietal pleura

R. bronch. v.

Br. of pulm. a.

Eparterial
bronchus

Post. pulm.
plexus

Int. mam. a.

Hyparterial
bronchus

Cut edge of peri-
cardial part of
parietal pleura

Lower r. pulm. v.

Inter-
costal v.,
a. and n.

Sulc. termin.
of r. atrium

Esophageal
plexus

Cut edge of
pericardium

R. atrium

Greater
splanchn. n.

Lesser
splanchn. n.

FIG. 92
Right view of mediastinum and root of the lung. (From Jones and Shepard, 1945.)

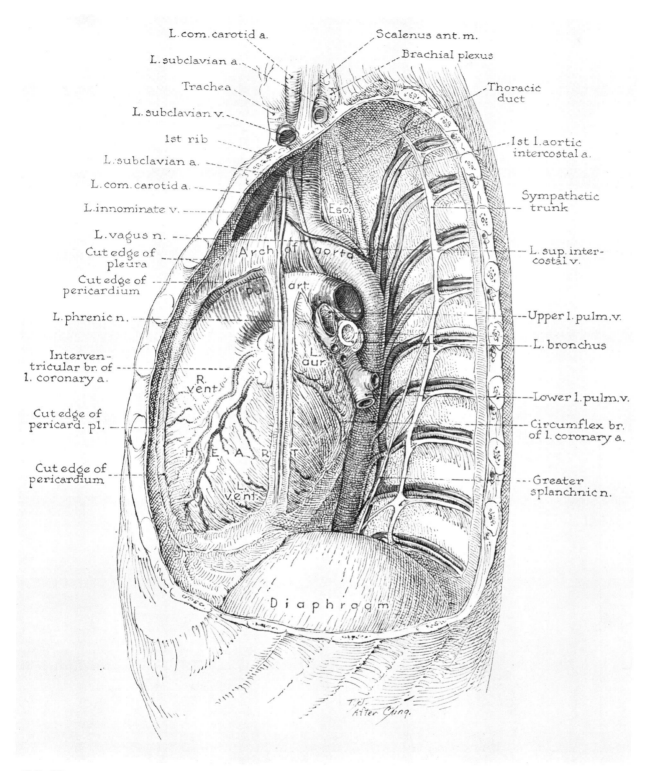

FIG. 93
Left view of mediastinum and root of the lung. (From Jones and Shepard, 1945.)

THE LUNG PEDICLE AND PULMONARY RESECTIONS   175

artery, and in front of the descending aorta, vagus nerve, and, more medially, the esophagus.

The constituents of each lung root are the pulmonary artery and principal bronchus of that side, the superior and inferior pulmonary veins, bronchial arteries and veins, pulmonary lymphatics, and pulmonary nerve plexus.

On each side, an anterior view shows the superior pulmonary vein (draining the upper lobe and on the right the middle lobe as well) anterior to and below the pulmonary artery (see Figs. 103, 106). It is only posteriorly that one can see the bronchus and the inferior pulmonary vein (see Figs. 94, 95, 105, 108). The pulmonary artery of each side lies anterior to the proximal part of the principal bronchus, but then courses differently on the two sides. On the right side (Fig. 94), it crosses the bronchus anterolaterally. At this point arise the upper lobe arteries and bronchus (the 'eparterial bronchus'). The artery then runs anterolateral to the intermediate and lower lobe bronchi but posterior to the middle lobe

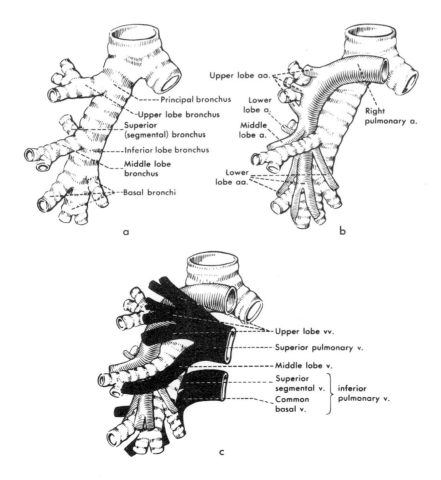

FIG. 94
Typical branching of chief bronchi and blood vessels, right lung. (From Hollinshead, 1956.)

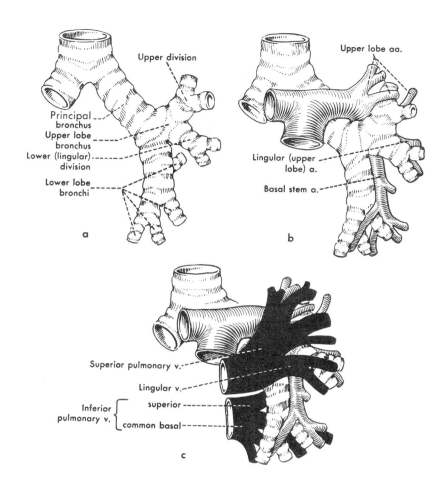

FIG. 95
Typical branching of chief bronchi and blood vessels, left lung. (From Hollinshead, 1956.)

bronchus. The left pulmonary artery (Fig. 95), beyond its initial portion, runs posterior to the upper lobe bronchus, and then assumes a position anterolateral to the lower lobe bronchus. The pulmonary arteries possess a substantial sheath in distinction to the thin sheath about the veins and the absence of any sheath about the bronchi.

Variations of the principal bronchi and pulmonary arteries are rare. A segmental bronchus of the right upper lobe may rarely arise directly from the trachea (Felson, 1960), but displacement of an otherwise normally distributed lobar bronchus probably does not occur. More peripherally there may occur proximal or distal displacement of segmental bronchi. 'Supernumerary' bronchi may occasionally be encountered; most of these are probably displaced subsegmental bronchi. The surgeon must carefully identify the distribution of any bronchus before dividing it.

In the rare abnormality of pulmonary sequestration, an aberrant pulmonary artery arises from the aorta or other

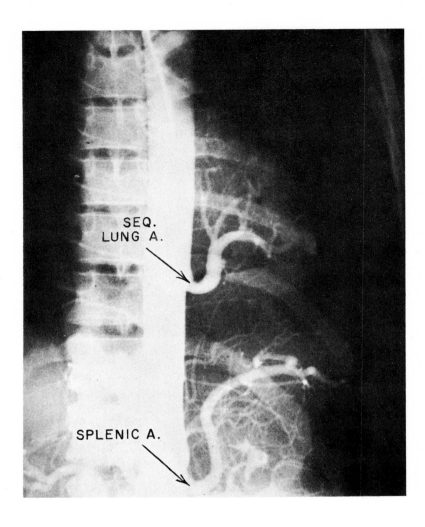

SEQ.
LUNG A.

SPLENIC A.

FIG. 96
Artery to sequestered lung.

systemic vessel to supply the sequestered lung tissue (Fig. 96). When this tissue lies embedded in the normal lung the condition is termed intralobar sequestration. The venous drainage in such instances is to a pulmonary vein, and there is continuity with a bronchus (Pryce, 1946; Burford and Ferguson, 1969). In the extralobar type, the abnormal pulmonary mass is separate from the normal lung tissue and possesses its own pleural covering. The mass is generally larger than that of the intralobar variety. It is most often located at the base of the left lung, and may be complicated by a hernia through the vertebrocostal foramen (of Bochdalek) (Valle and White, 1947; see Fig. 119). Venous drainage is to the azygos system, and there is no connection to a bronchus. The aberrant artery is often large, averaging 5 mm, passing through the vertebrocostal foramen. Surgical injury and severe hemorrhage have been reported.

The pulmonary veins are subject to variation at their termination. A common pulmonary vein formed by union of the superior and inferior trunks just outside of or within the pericardium has an incidence of 25 per cent on the left, but only 3 per cent on the right (Healey and Gibbon, 1950). More rarely, three pulmonary veins may enter the atrium from the right or left lung. The extent of the pulmonary veins lying free within the pericardial cavity may also vary considerably from the usual relationship shown in Figure 97. Most of the circumference of both left veins and the right superior vein is intrapericardial, but the left inferior vein may be almost entirely extrapericardial. These considerations are important for intrapericardial ligation of the veins or removal of portions of the atrium in cases of tumor extension or distal venous hemorrhage.

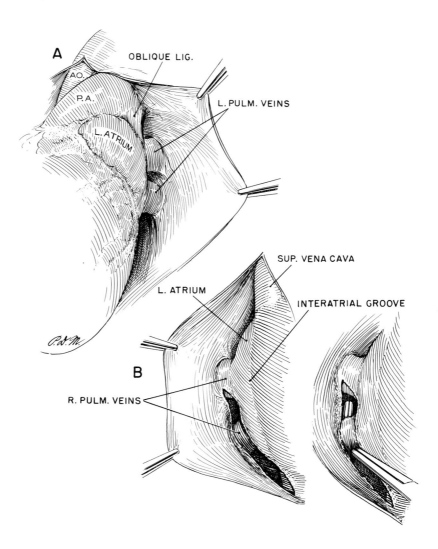

FIG. 97
Intrapericardial course of pulmonary veins.

7 *a*

The absence of valves within the pulmonary veins has suggested the possibility of retrograde flushing of the pulmonary arteries in operative pulmonary embolectomy (Gahagan and Manzor, 1965).

The bronchial arteries and veins have been considered in Chapter 7. Here we may note again that the bronchial artery usually lies posterior to the bronchus, although a left superior bronchial artery, or a trunk common to it, and the right bronchial artery may lie anterior to the initial part of the left principal bronchus. The bronchial arteries usually require separate ligation in pulmonary resection, particularly if they are enlarged.

MAJOR LYMPHATIC TRUNKS AND NODES

Figure 98 identifies the major lymphatic pathways. The lymphatic vessels are known to course as perivascular and peribronchial plexuses in the lung, some running first toward, then beneath the pleura. A few nodes are located within the

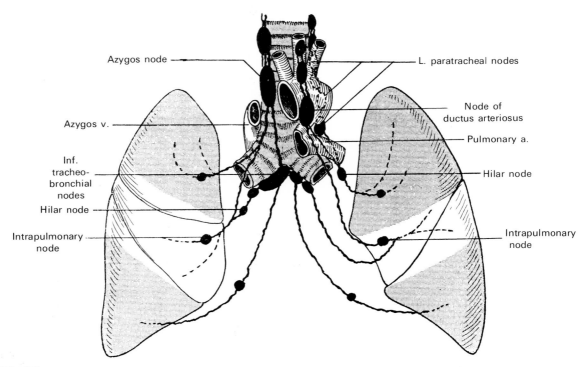

FIG. 98
Pulmonary lymphatics: overall view of regional drainage. (From Rouvière, 1932.)

lung near the hilum, and one or two are found in the pulmonary ligament. These drain into hilar nodes which connect with major regional nodes lying in relation to the principal bronchi and trachea. Subgroups of these nodes are called paratracheal, and the lowest of these are the lateral tracheobronchial nodes. Below the bifurcation of the trachea lie large inferior tracheobronchial, or carinal, nodes. Smaller pretracheal nodes tend to

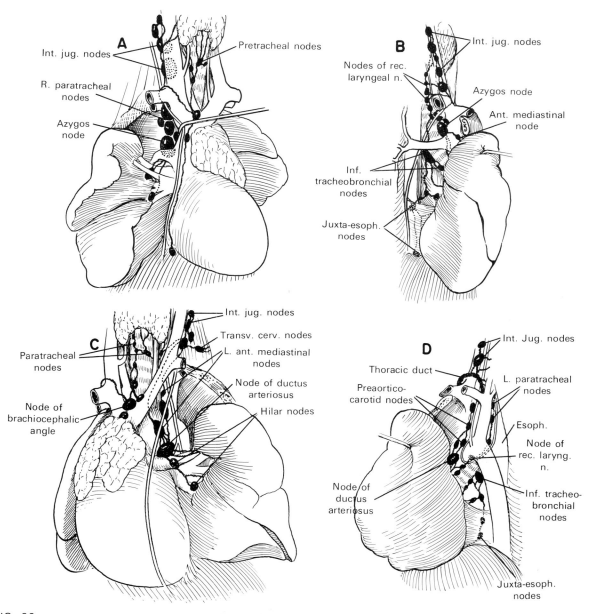

FIG. 99
Pulmonary lymphatics: anterior and posterior views of regional nodes, A and B, right, and C and D, left side. (After Rouvière, 1932.)

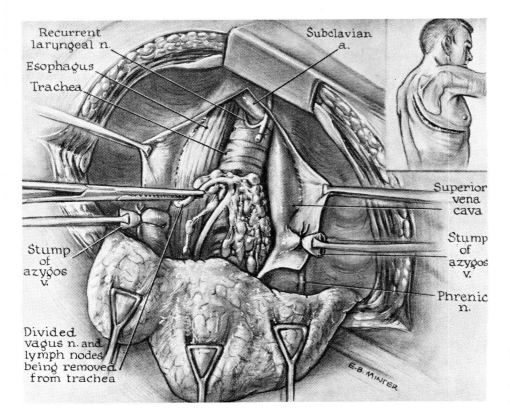

Recurrent laryngeal n.

Esophagus

Trachea

Subclavian a.

Superior vena cava

Stump of azygos v.

Phrenic n.

Stump of azygos v.

Divided vagus n. and lymph nodes being removed from trachea

E.B. MINTER

FIG. 100
Right radical pneumonectomy: early stage of dissection. (From Gibbon et al., 1955.)

form a single trunk on each side of the trachea; this trunk, when joined by parasternal efferents, is then called the bronchomediastinal trunk. On the left, this is one of the final tributaries of the thoracic duct. On the right, the bronchomediastinal trunk enters the jugular-subclavian venous junction alone or as the right lymph duct when it is joined by the right jugular and subclavian trunks.

The lymph vessels from the lung hilum to the major nodes along the bronchi and trachea course both anterior and posterior to the pulmonary arteries, veins, and bronchi, and cross the azygos and brachiocephalic veins and the aorta and its uppermost branches (Fig. 99). Certain nodes are fairly constant. One or two lie in the pulmonary ligament, the uppermost being large and located just below the inferior pulmonary vein, where it constitutes a guide to that vessel during surgery (see Figs. 105, 108). A node of the ductus arteriosus lies anteriorly at the junction of that structure and the aorta. The azygos node lies at the junction of the azygos and superior vena cava. The regional nodes of the lungs also receive lymph from the heart, trachea, and esophagus (see pp. 159 and 219).

The proximity of the upper pulmonary pathway to the internal jugular and subclavian lymph trunks and nodes allows retrograde spread of tumors or other diseases to nodes in other locations, such as the scalene node, where they are accessible for biopsy. This is discussed in Chapter 3, under Mediastinoscopy.

RADICAL PNEUMONECTOMY

Radical pneumonectomy implies *en bloc* removal, with the lung, of the regional lymph nodes about the trachea and its bifurcation. On the right, early division of the pleura and azygos vein gives access to the peritracheal tissues (Figs. 100, 101). The right pulmonary artery is shorter than the left and passes laterally behind the superior vena cava where, as previously noted in Figure 58, it is partially covered by parietal pericardium. Immediately lateral to the vena cava arises the

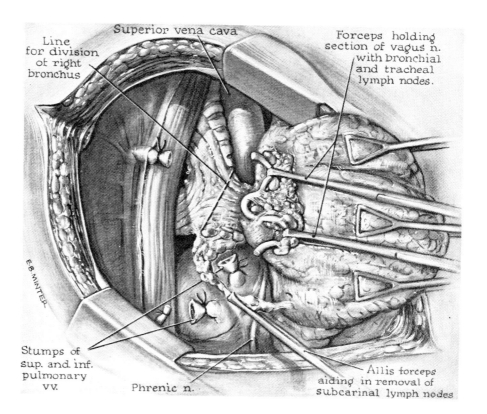

FIG. 101
Right radical pneumonectomy: late stage of dissection. (From Gibbon et al., 1955.)

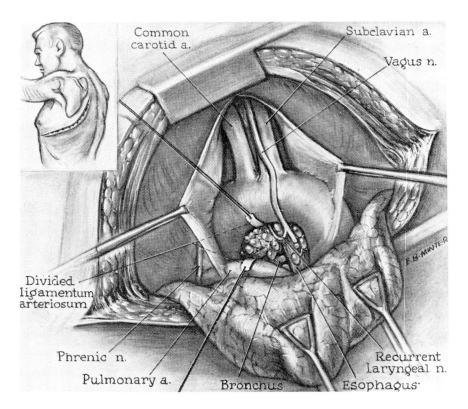

Common
carotid a.

Subclavian a.

Vagus n.

Divided
ligamentum
arteriosum

Phrenic n.

Pulmonary a.

Bronchus

Recurrent
laryngeal n.

Esophagus

FIG. 102

Beginning of a left radical pneumonectomy. The removal of fat and lymph nodes beneath the aortic arch is facilitated by traction on the stumps of the divided ligamentum arteriosum. The hilar structures are not yet clearly defined. (From Gibbon et al., 1955.)

truncus anterior, which is distributed to the apical and anterior segments of the upper lobe (see Fig. 103). The short length of the right pulmonary artery available between the vena cava and the origin of the truncus anterior usually makes it advisable to separately ligate the truncus and the artery beyond that branch. Additional length may be obtained by dissecting the pulmonary artery within the pericardium (see Fig. 58).

The left pulmonary artery arches above and posterolateral to the bronchus. Because of the greater length of the artery, it can generally be ligated proximal to its first branch (Figs. 102, 106).

If the veins are short or surrounded by tumor, they may be ligated within the pericardium. In some instances this may involve removal of some of the wall of the left atrium.

INTRAHILAR ANATOMY AND LOBAR OR SEGMENTAL RESECTION

The relationships of the major hilar structures have been discussed previously, in considering the lung root. Dissection at the hilum, either anteriorly, within the fissures, or posteriorly, reveals the pattern of further division of the pulmonary artery, vein, and bronchus. As already noted, there are frequent variations in the branching of these structures, and the surgeon must carefully identify individual branches before dividing them.

The first stage of dissection of the right hilum, from its anterior aspect, is shown in Figure 103. The pleura has been opened and reflected to expose the proximal portion of the pulmonary artery with its first branch, the truncus anterior. Immediately behind and above the artery is the bronchus, which is more easily palpated than visualized. Below and anterior to the artery is the superior pulmonary vein. The highest venous tributary drains the apical and part of the anterior segment; the lowest is the middle lobe vein. Between these are the posterior and inferior branches, which share a common trunk for a short distance. The posterior branch has come from deep within the hilum where it may frequently be encountered near the posterior segmental artery during dissection in the fissure.

In Figure 104 A the major fissure of the right lung has been opened widely to expose the interlobar course of the pulmonary artery as it lies anterior to the bronchus. The arteries to the posterior segment of the upper lobe, middle lobe, and the superior and basal segments of the lower lobe

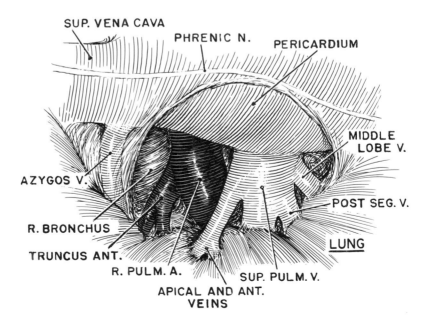

FIG. 103
Hilum of right lung: anterior view.

are exposed. There may be considerable variation from the pattern shown in this dissection. The posterior segmental artery, particularly, may arise from the main trunk at any point in its interlobar course or from the artery of the superior segment or of the middle lobe, or it may not be present as a separate vessel. The middle lobe or superior segment may be supplied by more than one branch. The posterior segmental vein (not evident in the specimen drawn) may often lie close by the origins of the superior segmental and middle lobe arteries and may be injured during exposure of these structures.

In Figure 104 B the superior and basal segmental arteries have been divided to expose the lower and middle lobe

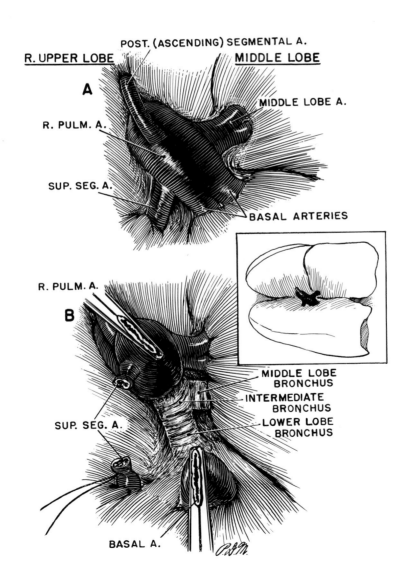

FIG. 104
Hilum of right lung: fissure view.

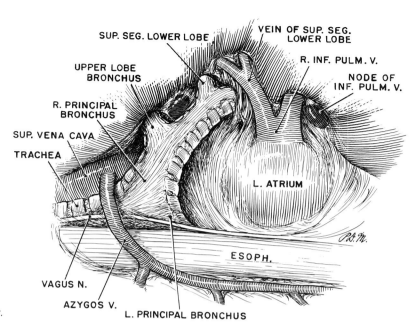

SUP. SEG. LOWER LOBE

VEIN OF SUP. SEG. LOWER LOBE

UPPER LOBE BRONCHUS

R. INF. PULM. V.

NODE OF INF. PULM. V.

R. PRINCIPAL BRONCHUS

SUP. VENA CAVA

TRACHEA

L. ATRIUM

ESOPH.

VAGUS N.

AZYGOS V.

L. PRINCIPAL BRONCHUS

FIG. 105
Hilum of right lung: posterior view.

bronchi. The origin of the superior segment bronchus lies slightly higher and posterior to the middle lobe bronchus in this specimen and would be seen by medial rotation of the bronchus.

The view of the posterior aspect of the right hilum shown in Figure 105 is more generous than that usually obtained at operation. It illustrates, however, what may be accomplished by anterior and medial traction upon the lung. The esophagus, trachea with adjacent vagus nerve, and superior vena cava receiving the azygos vein are seen. The tracheal bifurcation has been drawn into view and its relation to the left atrium may be appreciated. The inferior pulmonary vein is well visualized, with branches from the superior and basal segments of the lower lobe. The lymph node immediately below the inferior pulmonary vein is usually palpable high within the pulmonary ligament, and serves as a useful guide to the location of the inferior vein.

Dissection of the left hilum is begun from the anterior aspect as shown in Figure 106. The vagus nerve passes behind the hilar structures giving branches to the pulmonary plexus, some of which have been divided to better expose the pulmonary artery. The phrenic nerve lies anterior. The pleura has been opened to expose the pulmonary artery and superior pulmonary vein. The artery is the highest structure in the left hilum. The apicoposterior trunk is usually seen

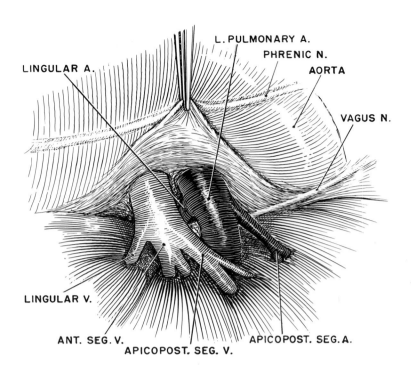

LINGULAR A.

L. PULMONARY A.

PHRENIC N.

AORTA

VAGUS N.

LINGULAR V.

ANT. SEG. V.

APICOPOST. SEG. V.

APICOPOST. SEG. A.

FIG. 106
Hilum of left lung: anterior view.

but the lingular artery is usually hidden beneath the vein. The branches of the superior vein are quite superficial and readily dissected in most instances.

Views of the structures within the fissure on the left are shown in Figure 107. Figure 107 A shows very well the close proximity of the left pulmonary artery and the aorta, which has made possible aorto-pulmonary anastomosis (Potts). Division of the segmental arteries (Fig. 107 B and C) exposes the bronchus. The lingular bronchus in this specimen is nearly as large as the lower lobe bronchus. The superior segment bronchus is not shown. It originates from the lower lobe bronchus posteriorly, at the level of the lingular bronchus (see Fig. 91 B).

Relationships in the posterior hilar dissection are shown in Figure 108. The pulmonary artery is the highest structure and in its descent passes posterior to the upper lobe bronchus. The posterior position of the inferior pulmonary vein is easily appreciated in this view. The recurrent laryngeal branch of the left vagus nerve is shown, but further dissection would be necessary to permit visualization of the ligamentum arteriosum around which it turns. Vagal branches to the posterior pulmonary plexus and to the esophagus are illustrated.

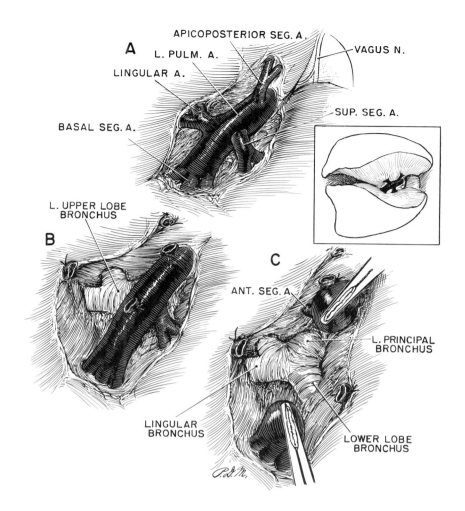

FIG. 107
Hilum of left lung: fissure view.

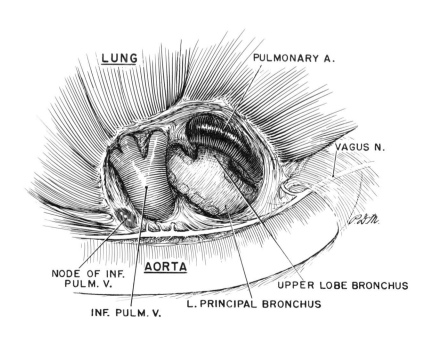

FIG. 108
Hilum of left lung: posterior view.

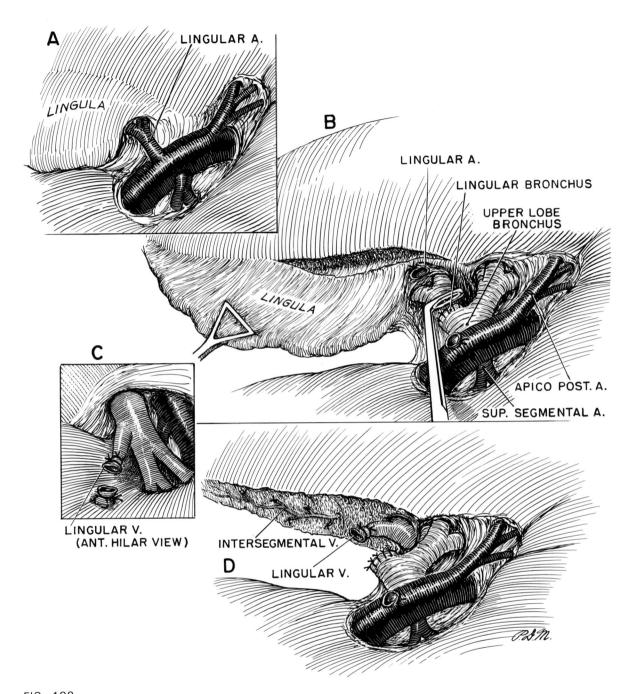

FIG. 109

Lingulectomy. A, B, and D show dissection in the fissure. In B, the segment is well demarcated after its bronchus is clamped. C illustrates the anterior approach to the lingular vein. In D, the lingula has been removed.

Figure 109 illustrates the anatomy of resection involving less than a lobe, in this instance the lingula, comprising two segments.

REFERENCES

Burford, T. H., and Ferguson, T. B.: Congenital Lesions of the Lungs and Emphysema. Chapter 18 *in* Surgery of the Chest, Gibbon, J. H., Jr., Sabiston, D. C., Jr., and Spencer, F. C., Eds., 2nd ed. Philadelphia, W. B. Saunders, 1969.

Felson, B.: Fundamentals of Chest Roentgenology. Philadelphia, W. B. Saunders, 1960.

Gahagan, T., and Manzor, A.: Anatomy of the pulmonary veins relative to removal of pulmonary emboli by retrograde flushing. Anat. Rec. 151:352, 1965 (abstract).

Gibbon, J. H., Jr., Stokes, T. L., and McKeown, J. J., Jr.: The surgical treatment of carcinoma of the lung. Amer. J. Surg. 89:484–493, 1955.

Healey, J. E., Jr., and Gibbon, J. H., Jr.: Intrapericardial anatomy in relation to pneumonectomy for pulmonary carcinoma. J. Thor. Surg. 19:864–874, 1950.

Hollinshead, W. H.: Anatomy for Surgeons. Vol. 2, The Thorax, Abdomen, and Pelvis. New York, Hoeber, 1956.

Jones, T., and Shepard, W. C.: A Manual of Surgical Anatomy. Philadelphia, W. B. Saunders, 1945.

Pryce, D. M.: Lower accessory pulmonary artery with intralobar sequestration of lung. A report of seven cases. J. Path. Bact. 58:457–467, 1946.

Rouvière, H.: Anatomie des lymphatiques de l'homme. Paris, Masson, 1932.

Valle, A. R., and White, M. L., Jr.: Subdiaphragmatic aberrant pulmonary tissue. Dis. Chest 13:63–68, 1947.

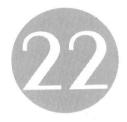

the trachea

EXPOSURE

The cervical portion of the trachea may easily be approached by a midline incision in the neck, parting the strap muscles in the relatively avascular median plane. With proper care to protect the laryngeal nerves on either side, the trachea may be freed well down into the superior mediastinum by this approach. The blood supply of the cervical trachea stems from three tracheo-esophageal branches of the inferior thyroid artery (Miura and Grillo, 1966) (Fig. 110).

Most tracheal injuries precipitated by the use of tracheostomy or endotracheal tubes may be repaired by tracheal reconstruction, using the cervical route. If further exposure of the trachea should be required, the incision can be extended in the midline and upper thoracic sternotomy performed. The incision is the same as that described previously for median sternotomy (Chapter 9), except for extension into the second, third, or fourth intercostal space on either side. Better exposure of the mediastinal trachea alone may be obtained through a right thoracotomy. The arch of the aorta prevents access to the trachea from the left side in most persons. Division of the terminal arch of the azygos vein and retraction of the superior vena cava allows excellent visualization of the right and posterolateral aspects of the trachea, its bifurcation, and the right bronchus. Anterior to the trachea

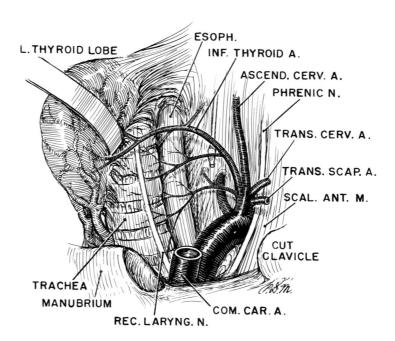

L. THYROID LOBE
ESOPH.
INF. THYROID A.
ASCEND. CERV. A.
PHRENIC N.
TRANS. CERV. A.
TRANS. SCAP. A.
SCAL. ANT. M.
CUT CLAVICLE
COM. CAR. A.
REC. LARYNG. N.
MANUBRIUM
TRACHEA

FIG. 110
Cervical tracheo-esophageal arteries.

are the brachiocephalic trunk and the left brachiocephalic vein. The vein may be divided if necessary.

RESECTION

The relative rigidity and blood supply of the trachea are two considerations of special importance in resection of this structure. Although Rob and Bateman (1949) deduced from studies of six fresh human cadavers that no more than 2 cm of trachea could be resected if primary anastomosis was to be accomplished, more recent studies have provided means for achieving considerably greater mobility. Barclay and associates (1957) described two steps to give additional mobility to the lower end of the trachea. These were (1) division of the left principal bronchus which is held in a caudal position by the arch of the aorta, and (2) mobilization of the root of the right lung by division of the pulmonary ligament. The left principal bronchus was then reimplanted into the intermediate bronchus (Fig. 111 **a**). The technique allowed primary reconstruction after removal of as much as 6 cm of trachea.

Grillo and associates (1964) advocated a third step, namely, freeing the pulmonary artery and veins from the

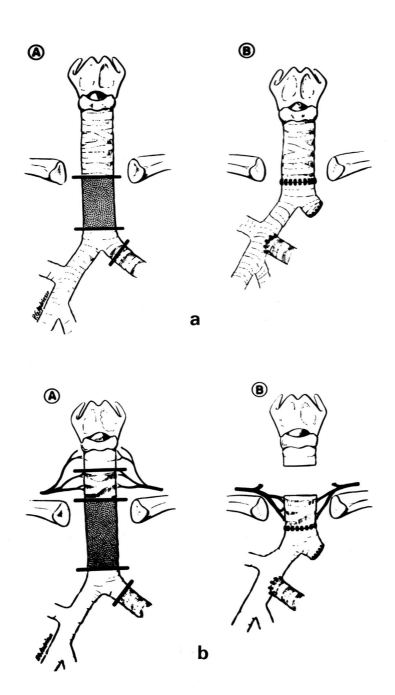

a

b

FIG. 111
Plans for resection of trachea. (From Grillo et al., 1964.)

pericardium. They analyzed the length of tracheal resection permitted by each of these steps in postmortem subjects. Mobilization of the right hilum gave a length averaging 3 cm, division of the left principal bronchus, 2.7 cm, and pericardial dissection, an additional 0.9 cm. The total resectable length averaged 6.4 cm (5.7 to 10 cm), or between 11 and 18 tracheal rings.

Grillo (1970) has emphasized that, with cervical hyperextension, the trachea may be mobilized through a collar incision to the bifurcation by anterior blunt dissection. If the trachea is then transected, blunt dissection posteriorly may complete the mobilization. This approach, although useful in benign disease, is not recommended for the treatment of malignant tumors. For these, partial or total sternotomy gives further exposure. Extension of the sternotomy incision into the right chest at the level of the fourth intercostal space provides access to the entire trachea, including its bifurcation. Dissection should be made in the loose areolar tissue surrounding the trachea rather than skeletonizing the tracheal cartilages. Denuding the cartilages may result in injury to the blood supply, and necrosis at the suture line.

The tendency of the trachea to retract into the thorax after division in the neck may allow a primary tracheal anastomosis in the mediastinum after a very long tracheal resection (Fig. 111 **b**). The cervical trachea may then be reconstructed with the use of prosthetic materials or by a tube fashioned from a skin graft supported by plastic rings. The displaced portion of the cervical trachea is mobilized by division of the upper branches of its blood supply from the inferior thyroid artery, while the lower branches are kept intact. No satisfactory circumferential prosthesis or tissue graft for reconstruction of the trachea within the mediastinum has yet been devised.

A comprehensive review of management of cancer of the trachea is that of Houston and associates (1969).

REFERENCES

Barclay, R. S., McSwan, N., and Welsh, T. M.: Tracheal reconstruction without the use of grafts. Thorax 12:177–180, 1957.

Grillo, H. C.: Surgery of the trachea. Current Problems in Surgery, July, 1970.

Grillo, H. C., Dignan, E. F., and Miura, T.: Extensive resection and reconstruction of mediastinal trachea without prosthesis or graft. An anatomical study in man. J. Thorac. Cardiovasc. Surg. 48:741–749, 1964.

Houston, H. E., Payne, W. S., Harrison, E. G., and Olsen, A. M.: Primary cancers of the trachea. Arch. Surg. 99:132–139, 1969.

Miura, T., and Grillo, H. C.: The contribution of the inferior thyroid artery to the blood supply of the human trachea. Surg. Gynec. Obstet. 123:99–102, 1966.

Rob, C. G., and Bateman, G. H.: Reconstruction of the trachea and cervical oesophagus. Preliminary report. Brit. J. Surg. 37:202–205, 1949.

SECTION 5

Thoracoabdominal Structures

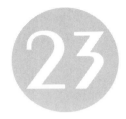

viscerAl topogRAphy
ANd exposures

SUBPHRENIC VISCERAL RELATIONSHIPS

The shape of the diaphragm is such that several abdominal viscera and some of the peritoneum rise up under each dome to be located within the bony confines of the thorax. These structures are capped peripherally by the costophrenic pleural sinuses, and that portion of each lung lying within the sinuses. The extent of this relationship is shown in Figures 112 to 115.

Beneath the right dome lies the liver in contact with the diaphragm over its bare area, and elsewhere separated by the right anterior and posterior ('subhepatic'—Boyd [1958]) subphrenic spaces (Figs. 116 and 117). Other viscera located here are the hepatic flexure of the colon, the right adrenal (suprarenal) gland, and the upper pole of the right kidney. A hepatic or a right posterior subhepatic abscess may be drained through the right costophrenic sinus and diaphragm.

In the concavity of the diaphragm, on the left side, lie a small portion of the liver, with the small left anterior subphrenic space in front of the left triangular ligament, and the left posterior subphrenic space behind it, partly anterior to the lesser omentum, partly in continuity with the omental

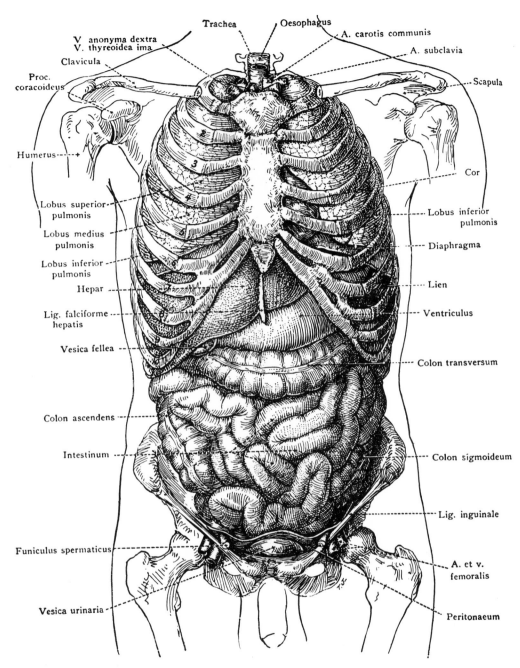

Trachea Oesophagus

V. anonyma dextra
V. thyreoidea ima   A. carotis communis

Clavicula   A. subclavia

Proc.
coracoideus   Scapula

Humerus   Cor

Lobus superior
pulmonis   Lobus inferior
                                       pulmonis

Lobus medius
pulmonis   Diaphragma

Lobus inferior
pulmonis   Lien

Hepar   Ventriculus

Lig. falciforme
hepatis   Colon transversum

Vesica fellea

Colon ascendens

Intestinum   Colon sigmoideum

                                      Lig. inguinale

Funiculus spermaticus   A. et v.
                                      femoralis

Vesica urinaria   Peritonaeum

FIG. 112
Relations of viscera to the skeleton: anterior view. (Medical Dept., U.S. Army, 1918.)

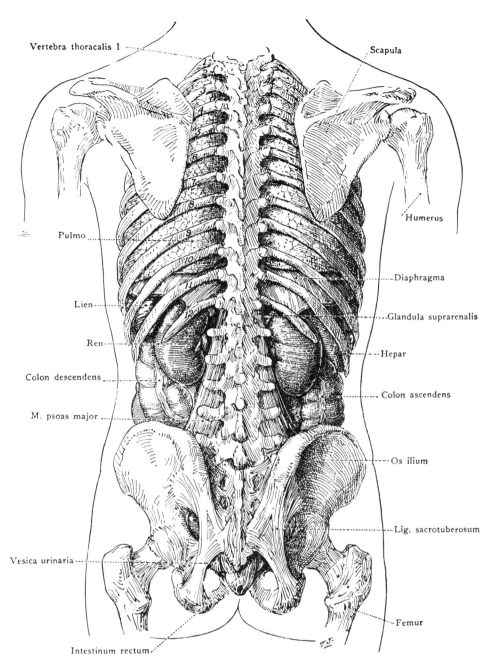

Vertebra thoracalis I

Scapula

Humerus

Pulmo

Diaphragma

Lien

Glandula suprarenalis

Ren

Hepar

Colon descendens

Colon ascendens

M. psoas major

Os ilium

Lig. sacrotuberosum

Vesica urinaria

Femur

Intestinum rectum

FIG. 113
Relations of viscera to the skeleton: posterior view. (Medical Dept., U.S. Army, 1918.)

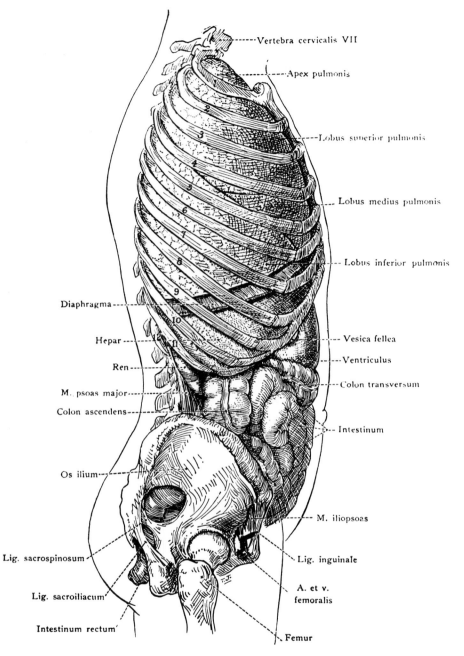

Vertebra cervicalis VII

Apex pulmonis

Lobus superior pulmonis

Lobus medius pulmonis

Lobus inferior pulmonis

Diaphragma

Hepar

Ren

M. psoas major

Colon ascendens

Vesica fellea

Ventriculus

Colon transversum

Intestinum

Os ilium

M. iliopsoas

Lig. sacrospinosum

Lig. inguinale

A. et v. femoralis

Lig. sacroiliacum

Intestinum rectum

Femur

FIG. 114
Relations of viscera to the skeleton: right lateral view. (Medical Dept., U.S. Army, 1918.)

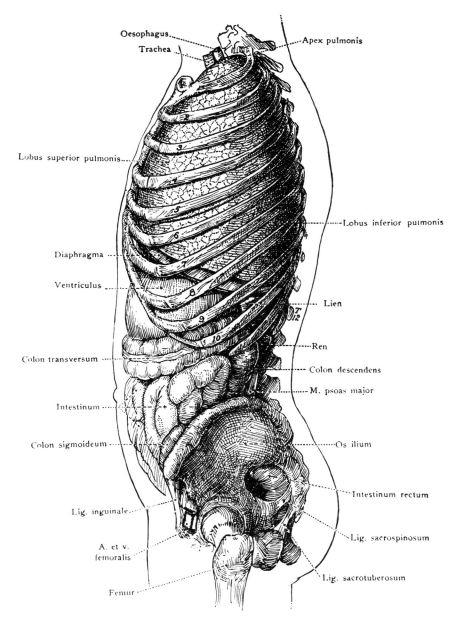

FIG. 115
Relations of viscera to the skeleton: left lateral view. (Medical Dept., U.S. Army, 1918.)

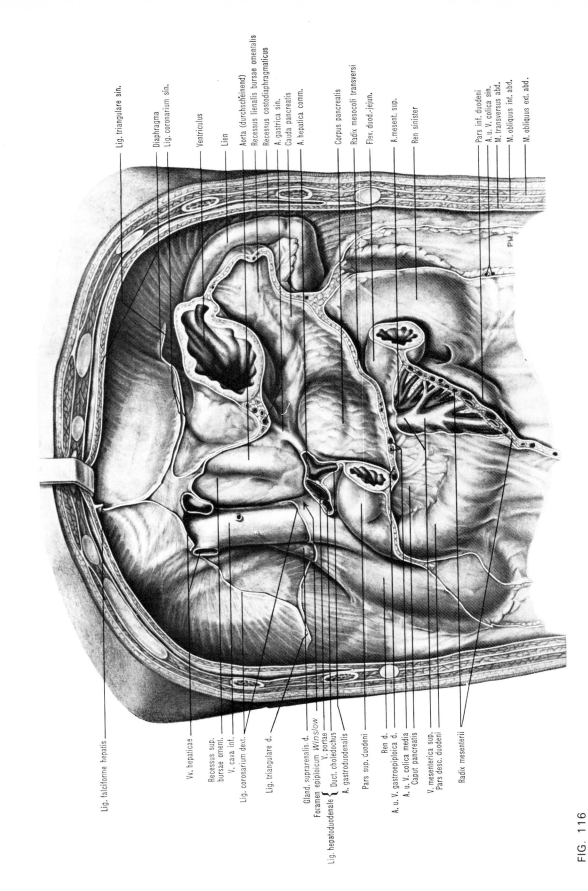

Lig. triangulare sin.

Diaphragma
Lig. coronarium sin.

Ventriculus

Lien

Aorta (durchscheinend)
Recessus lienalis bursae omentalis
Recessus costodiaphragmaticus
A. gastrica sin.
Cauda pancreatis
A. hepatica comm.

Corpus pancreatis

Radix mesocoli transversi

Flex. duod.-jejun.

A. mesent. sup.

Ren sinister

Pars inf. duodeni
A. u. V. colica sin.
M. transversus abd.
M. obliquus int. abd.
M. obliquus ext. abd.

Lig. falciforme hepatis

Vv. hepaticae

Recessus sup.
bursae oment.
V. cava inf.
Lig. coronarium dext.

Lig. triangulare d.

Gland. suprarenalis d.
Foramen epiploicum *Winslow*
V. portae
Lig. hepatoduodenale { Duct. choledochus
A. gastroduodenalis

Pars sup. duodeni

Ren d.
A. u. V. gastroepiploica d.
A. u. V. colica media
Caput pancreatis

V. mesenterica sup.
Pars desc. duodeni

Radix mesenterii

FIG. 116
Subphrenic peritoneal relationships. (From Töndury, 1965.)

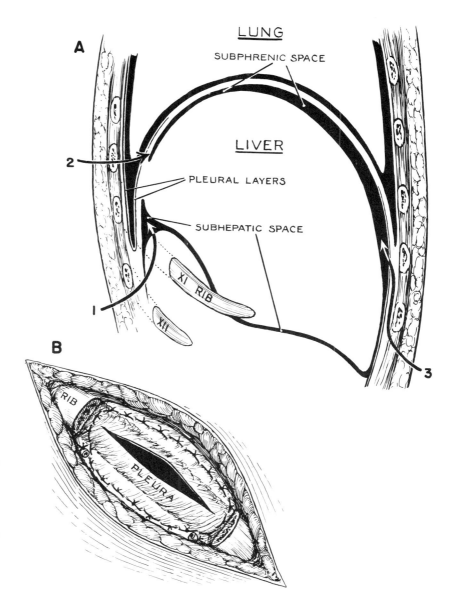

FIG. 117

Approaches to the subphrenic and subhepatic spaces. A. 1. Twelfth rib bed extraperitoneal route. 2. Transpleural route (more often used for intrahepatic abscess). 3. Anterior route. B. Obliteration of the costophrenic sinus for performance of transpleural drainage. (From Boyd, 1958.)

bursa. Other left subphrenic viscera are the stomach, the spleen (lying in the axis of the tenth rib), the splenic flexure of the colon, and, behind the omental bursa, the left adrenal gland and the upper pole of the left kidney.

THORACOABDOMINAL INCISIONS

Thoracoabdominal incisions may be planned to give simultaneous access to both the thoracic and the abdominal cavity or to allow a more ample exposure of the upper abdominal structures. Incisions may be both extrapleural and extraperitoneal—as for sympathectomy and splanchnicectomy (Fig. 14); or transpleural and transperitoneal—as for esophagectomy and esophagogastrostomy (see Figs. 129, 130), and for nephrectomy; or transpleural and extraperitoneal—as in Boyd's repair of hiatus hernia (p. 215) and in the sympathectomy of Linton *et al.* (Fig. 15).

In these exposures, the cavities may be opened by thoracotomy and incision solely of the diaphragm (see Figs. 129, 130), or by an incision of thorax and abdomen crossing the costal arch.

AVOIDANCE OF PHRENIC NERVE INJURY

An awareness of the major branching of the phrenic nerves on the diaphragm allows one to plan incisions with

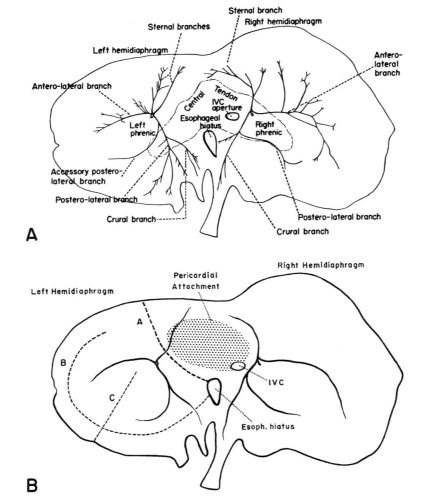

FIG. 118
Phrenic nerve branching (A) and diaphragmatic incisions (B). (After Merendino et al., 1956.)

a minimum of denervation of this structure. An excellent description is given by Merendino *et al.* (1956). The right phrenic nerve reaches the diaphragm just lateral to the aperture for the inferior vena cava, at times passing through the aperture alongside the vena cava. The left phrenic nerve enters the diaphragm more anteriorly, and lateral to the pericardium. On reaching the diaphragm, each nerve breaks up into three branches or groups of branches: sternal, anterolateral, and posterolateral (Fig. 118 A). These branches are often illustrated as being visible on the inferior surface of the diaphragm, but this is true in only about half of all subjects, and then for only short portions of their course.

Incisions producing least denervation are either radial in direction, pointing away from the parent nerve, or circumferential at the periphery (Fig. 118 B). Anterior incisions often cut the sternal branches, but only a small part of the muscle is affected. The superior phrenic branches of the pericardiacophrenic arteries, or the inferior phrenic arteries, may be divided. The crura are particularly vascular, containing large branches of the inferior phrenic arteries.

REFERENCES

Boyd, D. P.: The anatomy and pathology of the subphrenic spaces. Surg. Clin. N. Amer. 38:619–626, 1958.

Medical Department, United States Army: Manual of Surgical Anatomy, 1918. (No author or publisher named.)

Merendino, K. A., Johnson, R. J., Skinner, H. H., and Maguire, R. X.: The intradiaphragmatic distribution of the phrenic nerve with particular reference to the placement of diaphragmatic incisions and controlled segmental paralysis. Surgery 39:189–198, 1956.

Töndury, G.: Angewandte und topographische Anatomie, 3rd ed. Stuttgart, Georg Thieme, 1965.

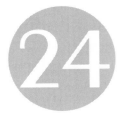

diapHRAqMATIC ANd HIATUS HERNIA

CONGENITAL DIAPHRAGMATIC HERNIA

A variety of hernias may result from the failure of development or of fusion of the elements that contribute to the formation of the diaphragm. The heaviest of these elements are the crura. The larger right crus arises from the anterior surface of the bodies of the first three or four lumbar vertebrae and the intervening discs. The left crus is shorter and thinner. The two crura decussate anterior to the aorta, the fibrous tissue crossing between them constituting the median arcuate ligament—a structure which is of variable thickness and which may be absent (Collis *et al.,* 1954). In at least half of all subjects there exists an 'intermediate crus' (Fig. 119), variably muscular or tendinous, arising from the vertebral bodies as low as the fourth lumbar.

Posterolaterally, the diaphragm takes origin from the lumbocostal arches or arcuate ligaments. The medial arcuate ligament extends from the medial crus to the transverse process of the first or second lumbar vertebra, arching anterior to the psoas muscle. The lateral arcuate ligament reaches from this transverse process to the lower edge of the twelfth rib, arching across the quadratus lumborum muscle. It is common to find a small triangular defect above the rib, due

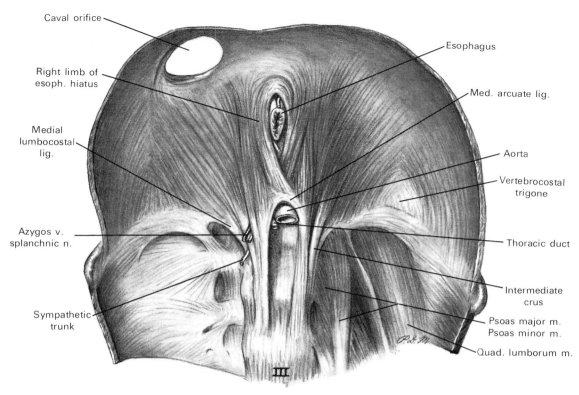

Caval orifice

Right limb of
esoph. hiatus

Medial
lumbocostal
lig.

Azygos v.
splanchnic n.

Sympathetic
trunk

Esophagus

Med. arcuate lig.

Aorta

Vertebrocostal
trigone

Thoracic duct

Intermediate
crus

Psoas major m.
Psoas minor m.

Quad. lumborum m.

III

FIG. 119
The diaphragm. The esophageal hiatus is most commonly formed from the right crus alone; in this case there is a contribution from the left. An 'intermediate crus' is present on one side or both in 50 per cent, and a psoas minor muscle in 60 per cent, of all subjects. (After Spalteholz, 1923.)

to lack of attachment of the muscle to the lateral lumbocostal arch. This is the foramen of Bochdalek, or the vertebrocostal foramen, or trigone. Here the retroperitoneal tissues, especially the kidney, lie in contact with the lower pleura. The commonest congenital hernias extend through this defect (Fig. 120). Extralobar pulmonary sequestration, when it occurs, is complicated by such a hernia in 30 per cent of cases (p. 178). In some instances there may be persistence of the embryonic pleuroperitoneal canal through this defect, with continuity of the two serous cavities.

Further laterally and anteriorly, the diaphragmatic origin continues from the inner surface of the lower sixth ribs and costal cartilages. On each side this costal origin meets the slip originating from the xiphoid. Failure of fusion at this meeting results in a small defect—the foramen of Morgagni, through which a hernia may form (Fig. 120). A peritoneal sac is said always to be present (Ravitch, 1964).

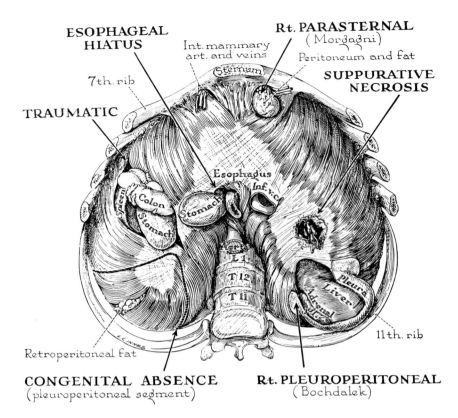

ESOPHAGEAL HIATUS
Int. mammary art. and veins
Rt. PARASTERNAL (Morgagni)
7th. rib
Peritoneum and fat
Sternum
SUPPURATIVE NECROSIS
TRAUMATIC
Esophagus
Inf. v.c.
Spleen
Colon
Stomach
Stomach
Aorta
L1
T12
T11
Pleura
Liver
Adrenal
11th. rib
Retroperitoneal fat
CONGENITAL ABSENCE
(pleuroperitoneal segment)
Rt. PLEUROPERITONEAL (Bochdalek)

FIG. 120
Types of diaphragmatic hernia. (From McVay, 1956.)

Large defects may exist in the more central parts of the muscle. The rare absence of the central tendon may be associated with congenital ventricular aneurysm or other cardiac or pericardial anomalies. It is postulated that a congenital defect in the diaphragm, or perforation by a pathologic process such as endometriosis, explains the occasional passage of blood or other fluid between the peritoneal and pleural cavities (Ganji and Vidrine, 1970).

HIATUS HERNIA

Operations for herniation of the stomach at the esophageal hiatus pose three major concerns for which anatomic answers may be sought. Two of these are common to all hernia surgery: the nature of the hernial sac, and the structures available for retention of the herniated organ after its reduction. The third, peculiar to hiatus hernia, is control of the peptic reflux that is characteristic of this disease.

Microscopic examination of the lower esophagus fails to demonstrate a particular muscle mass that can be called an intrinsic sphincter. However, the existence of a physiologic sphincter here seems well established by the feel of the esophagoscope, and by physiologic and roentgenologic evidence as summarized by Bockus (1963) (Fig. 121). As discussed below, the intrinsic sphincter appears to require, or at least is aided by, normal esophagogastric angulation in preventing reflux.

We are considerably indebted to Allison (1951) for elucidation of these questions. In most individuals, the esophageal hiatus is formed largely from the right crus of the diaphragm, which surrounds the esophagus with a right, or anterior, limb and a left, or posterior, limb (see Fig. 125). The left crus often contributes some muscle and rarely is the major source of the second limb of the hiatus. The muscular loop thus created sharply angulates the cardio-esophageal junction. This serves two functions: the first is to create an external and most significant sphincter which normally prevents reflux of gastric contents; the second is to force the cardia to adopt a position away from the long axis of the esophagus, so that intra-abdominal pressure pushes the stomach against the left dome of the diaphragm rather than through the hiatus. Allison likens this sphincteric action by angulation to that occurring at the ano-rectal junction (Fig. 122). The cardio-esophageal angulation is lost in hiatus hernia, the hiatus being stretched posteriorly by separation of its two limbs. According to Hill (1967), even more

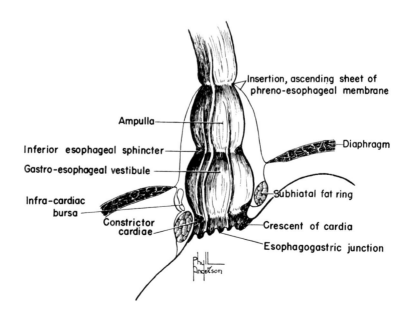

FIG. 121
Physiologic divisions of the distal esophagus. The 'infracardiac bursa' is said to be an inconstant derivative of the embryonic pleuroperitoneal canal. (From Palmer, 1952, based on Lerche, 1950.)

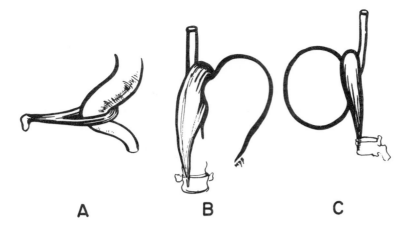

FIG. 122
Role of muscle sling in sphincteric function. (From Allison, 1951.) A. The puborectalis sling around the anorectal junction. B. The hiatal muscle sling around the esophagogastric junction. C. The hiatal sling in lateral view.

important in maintaining the angulation of the junction and its retention below the diaphragm is its anchorage by the heavy posterior part of the phreno-esophageal fascia (see below). The proximity of the central tendon anteriorly apparently prevents such a separation there. The structure that herniates upward through the patulous hiatus is the stomach, its long axis now being aligned with that of the esophagus (Fig. 123 B).

Such a hernia is a sliding hernia, with a partial sac on the left anterolateral aspect. The sac is so located since it is only on the left anterolateral aspect that the peritoneum is related to the esophagogastric junction.

The second and less common type of hiatus hernia is the para-esophageal hernia (Fig. 123 C). In this type the initial herniating part is a sac of peritoneum, again originating on the left anterior aspect of the esophagogastric junction, for the reason already given. The contents of the sac are the stomach and occasionally also a portion of the colon. The cardio-esophageal angle may be intact.

Fascial relationships are important in repair of hiatus hernia. The endo-abdominal fascia, here as throughout the abdomen, lines the parietes extraperitoneally. Again, as elsewhere, there is a continuity between the endo-abdominal fascia and the fascia propria of a viscus passing through the wall. The structure produced by attachment of the fascia on the under surface of the diaphragm to the esophageal fascia has been termed the phreno-esophageal fascia (Fig. 123 A). Its relationships in sliding and para-esophageal hiatus hernias are shown in Figure 123 B and C. The

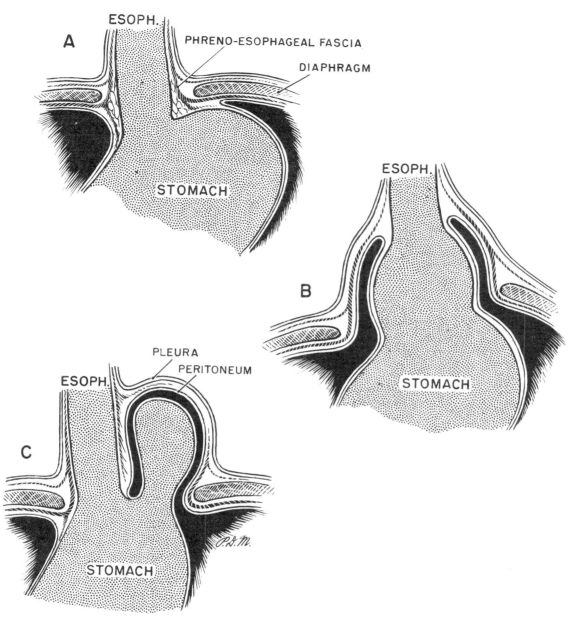

FIG. 123

Varieties of hiatus hernia. The disposition of structures at the esophageal hiatus are shown for the normal in A, in a sliding hernia in B, and in a para-esophageal hernia in C.

phreno-esophageal fascia is used in repositioning the esophagus, or the cardia, below the diaphragm after the hiatus hernia is reduced. It is thin anteriorly, where it may defy definition, but heavy posteriorly, as it extends down to the decussation of the crura anterior to the aorta.

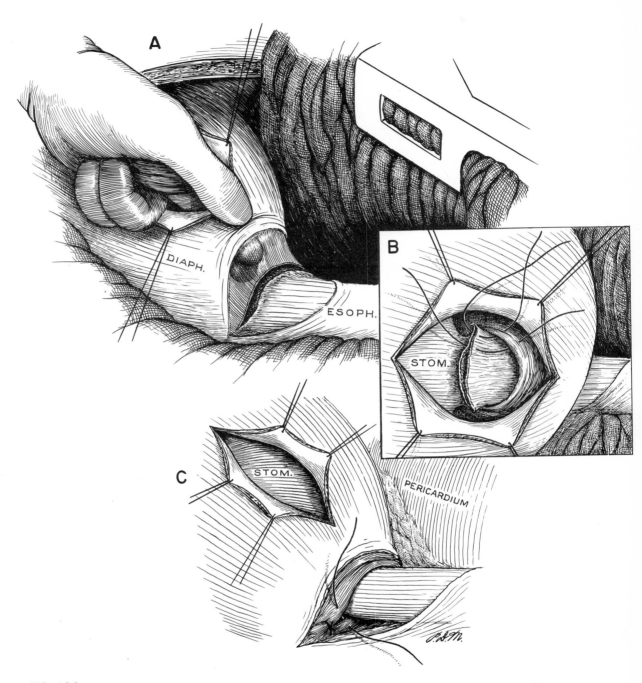

FIG. 124

Thoracic repair of esophageal hiatus hernia. (After Allison, 1951.) A. The pleura has been opened over the hiatus. With the fingers in the sac, the phreno-esophageal fascia has been incised. The peritoneum of the sac, presenting anterior to the esophagus, is still intact.   B. The esophagogastric junction has been pulled into the abdomen. The upper edge of the cut phreno-esophageal fascia is being sutured to the inferior surface of the hiatus.   C. The hiatus is narrowed behind the esophagus.

Operations for Hiatus Hernia

The major steps in the transthoracic operation are presented by Allison (1951) (Fig. 124). Access is by a low left thoracotomy. An incision in the diaphragm (avoiding the phrenic branches anteriorly) (Fig. 118 B) gives entrance to the sac from below to aid in the dissection. After the hiatus is narrowed posteriorly, the transdiaphragmatic view allows low fixation of the upper edge of the divided phreno-esophageal fascia to the inferior surface of the diaphragm. This step aids in accentuating the cardio-esophageal angle. Boyd (1964) describes three maneuvers to relax the limbs of the hiatus in order to perform the operation from above without incising the diaphragm: (1) The pleura is extensively incised and elevated. (2) The pericardium is separated from the diaphragm from the left phrenic nerve to the inferior vena cava. (3) The two limbs of the hiatus can now be separated to create a space adequate to allow the low fixation of the

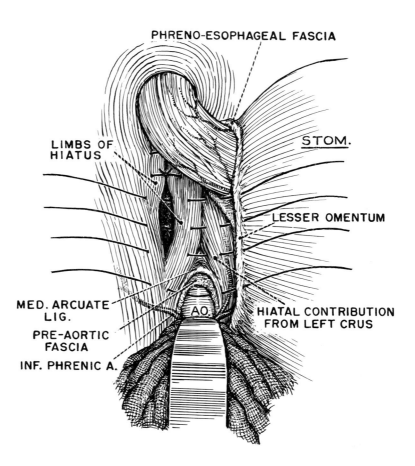

FIG. 125
Abdominal repair of hiatus hernia.
(After Hill, 1967.)

8

cut phreno-esophageal fascia and subsequent suturing of the hiatus behind the esophagus.

Vagotomy over the exposed supradiaphragmatic esophagus is sometimes added in instances of concomitant peptic ulcer. This maneuver is not likely to denervate the sphincter mechanism of the lower esophagus, since the vagal branches to this region are given off just below the lung roots (Hovelacque, 1927).

The repair of hiatus hernia from below involves an approach by division of the left triangular ligament so that the left lobe of the liver can be retracted anteriorly and to the right. The same structures are utilized as when the repair is done from above, except that the sutures which anchor the cardio-esophageal angle are also placed in the left crus, median arcuate ligament, and periaortic fascia (Hill, 1967) (Fig. 125).

The repair of a para-esophageal hernia, once the sac is open and the hernia reduced, is much the same as that of a sliding hernia.

REFERENCES

Allison, P. R.: Reflux esophagitis, sliding hiatal hernia, and the anatomy of repair. Surg. Gynec. Obstet. 92:419–431, 1951.

Bockus, H. L.: Gastroenterology, 2nd ed. Vol. 1, Examination of the Patient—The Stomach and the Esophagus. Philadelphia, W. B. Saunders, 1963.

Boyd, D. P.: The Transthoracic Repair of Esophageal Hiatus Hernia. Chapter 28 in Hernia, Nyhus, L. M., and Harkins, H. N., Eds. Philadelphia, J. B. Lippincott, 1964.

Collis, J. L., Kelly, T. D., and Wiley, A. M.: Anatomy of the crura of the diaphragm and the surgery of hiatus hernia. Thorax 9:175–189, 1954.

Ganji, H., and Vidrine, A., Jr.: Ectopic pregnancy presenting as hemothorax. Amer. J. Surg. 120:807–809, 1970.

Hill, L. D.: An effective operation for hiatal hernia. An eight year appraisal. Ann. Surg. 166:681–692, 1967.

Hovelacque, A.: Anatomie des nerfs craniens et rachidiens et du système grand sympathique. Paris, Doin, 1927.

Lerche, W.: The Esophagus and Pharynx in Action. A Study of Structure in Relation to Function. Springfield, Charles C Thomas, 1950.

McVay, C. B.: Hernia. Chapter 19 *in* Christopher's Textbook of Surgery, Davis, L., Ed., 6th ed. Philadelphia, W. B. Saunders, 1956.

Palmer, E. D.: The Esophagus and Its Diseases. New York, Hoeber, 1952.

Ravitch, M. M.: Congenital Diaphragmatic Hernia. Chapter 34 *in* Hernia, Nyhus, L. M., and Harkins, H. N., Eds. Philadelphia, J. B. Lippincott, 1964.

Spalteholz, W.: Hand-Atlas of Human Anatomy. Edited and translated from the seventh German edition by Barker, L. F. 4th ed. in English. Philadelphia, J. B. Lippincott, 1923.

RESECTION AND REPLACEMENT
of the esophagus

GENERAL CONSIDERATIONS

The design of operation for resection and replacement of the esophagus is influenced by three considerations.

1. *Course of the Esophagus.* In the neck and at its termination, the esophagus lies somewhat to the left of the midline. Its location, therefore, and the frequent use of the stomach to replace it dictate that many approaches will be made from the left. In the upper thorax, the barrier of the aortic arch has led to some right-sided approaches for this segment.

2. *Blood Supply.* The blood vessels of the esophagus, mostly shared with those of contiguous organs, are meager at the upper and lower ends of the thoracic portion (Figs. 40, 41), so that anastomosis is often performed in the neck rather than in the apex of the thorax.

3. *Pattern of Carcinoma.* When carcinoma involves the cervical segment, operation may be extended to remove the trachea or hypopharynx and the regional nodes (internal jugular, subclavian), since their resection is feasible. Carcinoma of the abdominal segment either spreads to the cardia of the stomach or arises there. Its lymphatic spread is to the nodes about the stomach. For these reasons, operations on the abdominal segment usually include a partial or com-

plete gastrectomy with removal of gastric lymph nodes (Hood and Kirklin, 1953). In some instances the resection is extended to remove the spleen, the distal pancreas, and the omentum. The thoracic esophagus, when the seat of carcinoma that has spread to contiguous structures, is usually considered unresectable. Adherent posterior mediastinal nodes and the nodes of the pulmonary ligament are usually removed, but no *en bloc* removal is attempted of the tracheobronchial and pulmonary hilar nodes which also receive esophageal lymph drainage.

STRUCTURES EMPLOYED FOR BYPASS GRAFTING OR REPLACEMENT

Central to current operations on the esophagus is the ability to bypass or replace the organ by a pedicled portion of the gastrointestinal tract, the Roux loop. Ten years after Roux introduced his 'gastroentérostomie en Y' (1897), he reported (1907) on the bypassing of the obstructed esophagus by a pedicled loop of jejunum laid subcutaneously from an anastomosis with the stomach to a premanubrial stoma (Fig. 126).

Currently the stomach, pedicled on its right gastric and right gastroepiploic arteries, is most frequently employed after resection of the thoracic esophagus. It is mobilized by dividing the left gastric, left gastroepiploic, and short gastric arteries, and the peritoneal ligaments in which they run, carefully preserving the arches which connect them to the two right-sided arteries. Garlock (1971) also divides the right paraduodenal peritoneum (the Kocher maneuver) to add mobility and prevent axial rotation and kinking of the duodenum. The stomach so mobilized can usually reach the highest part of the thoracic esophagus for anastomosis.

When gastrectomy is required the jejunum in a 'Roux en Y' loop can be anastomosed to the upper esophagus. Nakayama (1971) has utilized presternal (subcutaneous) position of the esophageal replacement for high thoracic carcinoma as well, obviating future obstruction of an orthotopic replacement that may result from recurrence of carcinoma in the old esophageal bed.

In very high lesions the stomach may not reach high

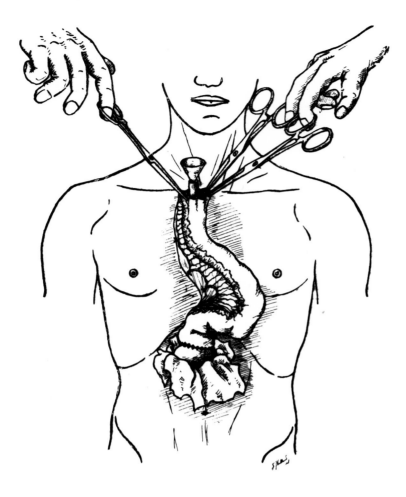

FIG. 126
*Esophageal bypass by subcutaneous
pedicled jejunogastrostomy. (From
Roux, 1907.)*

enough for an anastomosis to the cervical esophagus. In such cases the esophagus may be replaced by a pedicled loop of jejunum, or of terminal ileum–cecum and ascending and right half of the transverse colon, pedicled on the middle colic artery (Mahoney and Sherman, 1954; Petrov, 1964) (Fig. 127).

Anatomic limitations in the vascular arcades of the small intestine may make the length of jejunum available shorter than a colonic graft. Beck and Baronofsky (1960), in an anatomic study, found that the 'right colon' (the large bowel to the right of the mid transverse colon) was of inadequate length for such an anastomosis. The 'left colon' (from mid transverse colon to the sigmoid between the first and second sigmoid arteries) was always adequate in length. The practical length of the bowel depended on the length of the marginal artery. They found that a frequent narrowing of the marginal artery near the splenic flexure could be overcome by preserving the secondary arcade formed by the bifurcation of the left colic artery. Variations in the vascular pattern, particularly with regard to the middle colic artery, can reduce the adequacy of the pedicle of either the right or the left half of the colon.

The occasional inadequacy of the blood vessels in long grafts of either the jejunum or the colon has been overcome by vascular anastomosis. Thus, Longmire (1947) utilized a Roux loop of jejunum with anastomosis of the jejunal vessels to the internal thoracic, secured by resection of two left costal cartilages and rib segments. Nakayama (1971) has anastomosed the vessels of free segments of stomach, jejunum, or colon to some branches of the subclavian artery and adjacent vein. Similar free grafts of jejunum or colon with local vascular anastomoses have been used to replace the cervical esophagus (Jurkiewicz, 1965; Chrysopathis, 1966) (Fig. 128).

Bypass grafts without esophageal resection are often employed for benign stricture. Thoracotomy is avoided by placing the graft in a presternal or retrosternal tunnel, anastomosing above to the cervical esophagus and below to the

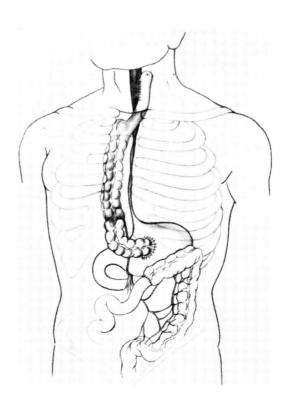

FIG. 127
Esophageal bypass by retrosternal pedicled esophago-ileocolic-gastrostomy. (From Petrov, 1964.)

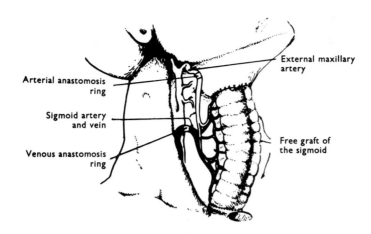

FIG. 128
Replacement of cervical esophagus by free graft of sigmoid colon with vascular anastomosis. (From Chryso-pathis, 1966.)

stomach or jejunum. Gavriliu (1971) used a tubular graft fashioned from the greater curvature of the stomach pedicled on the cardiac end. Petrov (1964) utilized the terminal ileum and right half of the colon, pedicled on the middle colic artery and mesenteric arcades (Fig. 127).

LOW THORACIC ESOPHAGECTOMY AND ESOPHAGOGASTRIC ANASTOMOSIS

The thoracic approach for low esophagectomy and esophagogastric anastomosis (Figs. 129 and 130) is by a left thoracotomy performed as high as the fifth or as low as the eighth rib or intercostal space, often with section of adjacent ribs or cartilages. The abdomen may be entered by sectioning the costal arch and cutting across the rectus muscle to or beyond the midline. Because of difficulty in the healing of cartilage, most surgeons prefer to enter the abdomen through the diaphragm. Merendino (1971) incises the diaphragm with an anterior radial incision located medial to the phrenic nerve and extended to the esophageal hiatus (Fig. 118 B). This divides the small sternal branch of the phrenic nerve.

The esophagus is exposed by detaching the pulmonary ligament anterior to the descending aorta. Juxta-esophageal nodes, including those of the ligament and the node of the inferior pulmonary vein, are taken with the esophagus. As the esophagus is freed, the veins and arteries entering its posterior surface are divided. The esophagus is thus withdrawn from the right pleura and the left atrium anteriorly, and the azygos vein, thoracic duct, and aorta behind (Fig. 18). The vagus nerves are removed with the esophagus when the operation is done for cancer. Vagal branches to the posterior pulmonary plexuses are divided, and the trunks are sectioned at the level of the aortic arch, the left below the origin of its recurrent laryngeal branch.

Above the aortic arch, division of the pleura and the left superior intercostal vein reveals the upper thoracic esopha-

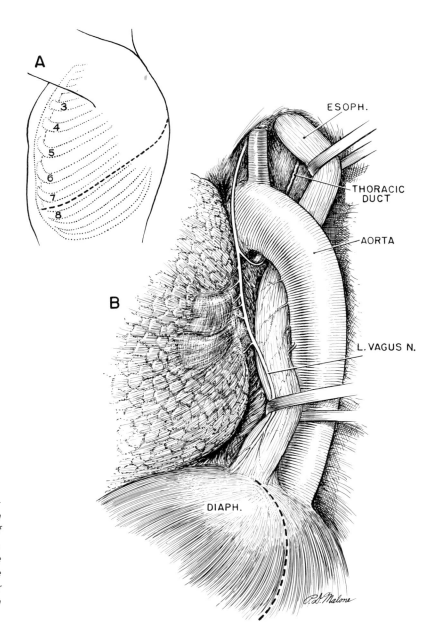

FIG. 129
Thoracic esophagectomy. A. Incision. The thorax is entered through the seventh intercostal space, and if necessary for a high anastomosis, separately through the third. B. The esophagus has been mobilized. The stomach or other viscus used for anastomosis is approached through the diaphragm.

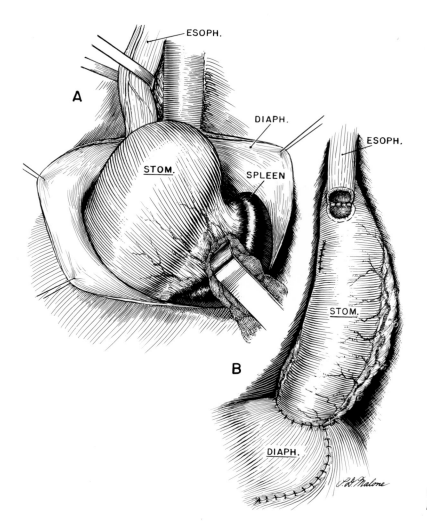

FIG. 130
Esophagogastrostomy.

gus. The left recurrent laryngeal nerve lies in the groove between it and the trachea. The thoracic duct here lies on its left lateral border. Dissection beneath the arch allows division of the esophageal branches of the bronchial arteries. Once these are divided, the only arteries remaining are those descending from the tracheo-esophageal branches of the inferior thyroid artery (see Fig. 110). Avascular necrosis of the anastomotic suture line to be placed here may result unless only a short esophageal stump is left behind (Sweet, 1946).

The stomach is now mobilized as described above, the esophagus is sectioned at the stomach, and the esophago-gastric anastomosis is performed (Fig. 130).

HIGH THORACIC ESOPHAGECTOMY AND
RIGHT-SIDED APPROACHES

The upper esophagus may be removed by a left thoracotomy as described, but a right-sided approach is also practiced. As Lewis (1946) said, only the azygos vein needs to be divided to give approach to the whole course of the esophagus. Dissection into the abdomen can be carried out through a separate or a combined incision. Nakayama originally (1954) cut across the right costal cartilages, but later (1971) advised against it because of difficulty in healing. The anastomosis of stomach or bowel is done on the right. These structures are brought up by dilating the esophageal hiatus or by making a separate incision in the diaphragm. Such an incision will pass through the right crus, which

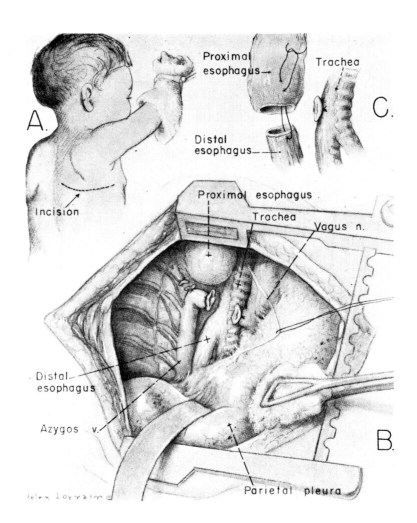

FIG. 131
Extrapleural approach to esophageal atresia and tracheo-esophageal fistula. (From Bigger, 1953). The vagus nerve is a useful guide to the atrophic lower end of the esophagus.

surrounds the esophageal hiatus. Care must be taken to avoid injury to the thoracic duct and the azygos vein, which lie beneath the crus.

EXTRAPLEURAL APPROACHES TO THE THORACIC ESOPHAGUS

The first transpleural resection of the esophagus was done by Franz Thorek of New York in 1913 (Lilienthal, 1925). For the next two or three decades, however, extrapleural approach by posterior mediastinotomy was more widely practiced, as by Lilienthal. The extrapleural approach is still useful for removal of a foreign body and drainage (see Fig. 20). It is also practiced as an alternative to transpleural operation for esophageal atresia in children with or without tracheo-esophageal fistula (Fig. 131).

REFERENCES

Beck, A. R., and Baronofsky, I. D.: A study of the left colon as a replacement for the resected esophagus. Surgery 48:499–509, 1960.

Bigger, I. A.: Congenital Atresia of the Esophagus. Chapter 39 *in* Operative Surgery, Horsley, G. W., and Bigger, I. A., Eds., ed. 6, vol. 1. St. Louis, Mosby, 1953.

Chrysopathis, P.: The contribution of vascular surgery to oesophageal replacement. Brit. J. Surg. 53:122–126, 1966.

Cooper, P., Ed.: The Craft of Surgery, ed. 2, vol. 1. Boston, Little, Brown and Company, 1971.

Garlock, J. H.: Esophagectomy for Carcinoma. Chapter 31 *in* Cooper, P., *op. cit.* (1971).

Gavriliu, D.: Procedure for Replacement of the Esophagus. Chapter 36 *in* Cooper, P., *op. cit.* (1971).

Hood, R. T., Jr., and Kirklin, J. W.: Usefulness of the abdomino-thoracic incision. Surg. Clin. N. Amer. 33:1447–1455, 1953.

Jurkiewicz, M. J.: Vascularized intestinal graft for reconstruction of the cervical esophagus and pharynx. Plast. Reconstr. Surg. 36:509–517, 1965.

Lewis, I.: The surgical treatment of carcinoma of the oesophagus, with special reference to a new operation for growths of the middle third. Brit. J. Surg. 34:18–31, 1946.

Lilienthal, H.: Thoracic Surgery. Philadelphia, W. B. Saunders, 1925.

Longmire, W. P., Jr.: A modification of the Roux technique for antethoracic esophageal reconstruction. Anastomosis of the mesenteric and internal mammary blood vessels. Surgery 22:94–100, 1947.

Mahoney, E. B., and Sherman, C. D., Jr.: Total esophagoplasty using intrathoracic right colon. Surgery 35:937–946, 1954.

Merendino, K. A.: Jejunal Interposition Operation. Chapter 38 *in* Cooper, P., *op. cit.* (1971).

Nakayama, K.: Approach to midthoracic esophageal carcinoma for its radical surgical treatment. Surgery 35:574–589, 1954.

Nakayama, K.: Carcinoma of the Thoracic and Cervical Esophagus. Chapter 33 *in* Cooper, P., *op. cit.* (1971).

O'Shaughnessy, L., and Raven, R. W.: Surgical exposure of the oesophagus. Brit. J. Surg. 22:365–377, 1934.

Petrov, B. A.: Retrosternal artificial esophagus created from colon. 100 operations. Surgery 55:520–523, 1964.

Roux: De la gastro-entérostomie. Rev. gynécol. chir. abdom. 1:67–122, 1897.

Roux: L'oesophago-jéjuno-gastrostomose, nouvelle opération pour rétrécissement infranchissable de l'oesophage. Sem. méd. 27:37–40, 1907.

Sweet, R. H.: Carcinoma of the midthoracic esophagus. Its treatment by radical resection and high intrathoracic esophagogastric anastomosis. Ann. Surg. 124:653–666, 1946.

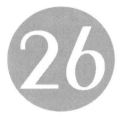

the thoracic duct

USUAL PATTERN OF THE THORACIC DUCT
AND ITS TRIBUTARIES

In about 90 per cent of individuals, the thoracic duct ,tarts as a 3- to 5-mm-wide continuation of the cisterna chyli, between the right crus of the diaphragm and the upper abdominal aorta, on the bodies of the first and second lumbar vertebrae (Fig. 132). It ascends through the aortic hiatus, between the aorta and azygos vein. The duct remains a right-sided structure in the lower posterior mediastinum, but turns to the left behind the esophagus over the fifth vertebral body (see Fig. 18). In its further ascent it lies on the left posterior border of the esophagus adjacent to the left pleura.

The thoracic duct enters the neck behind the left carotid sheath. Figure 133 shows its terminal portion running in front of the subclavian artery and its branches, the scalenus anterior muscle, and the phrenic nerve. It terminates in the angle of junction of the left internal jugular and subclavian veins, or, rarely, in the vertebral vein.

The major trunks drained by the thoracic duct are those that enter the cisterna chyli below and those that join it at its termination. The cisterna receives a single anterior intestinal trunk, from the territory of the celiac and superior mesenteric arteries, and two para-aortic or lumbar trunks from the

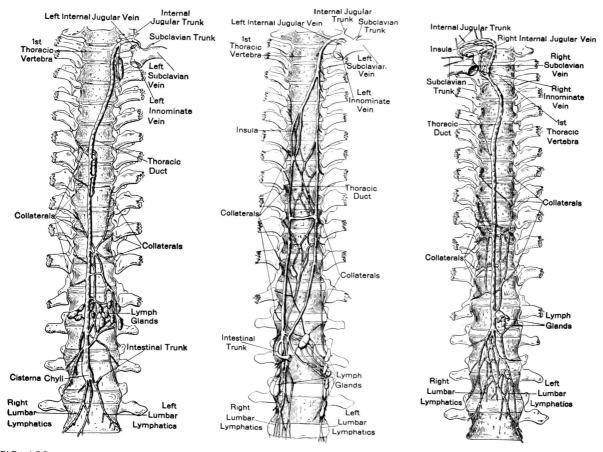

FIG. 132

Variations of the thoracic duct. Left, a duct conforming to the usual description. Middle, absence of a cisterna chyli, and duplication of much of the course of the duct. Right, absence of a cisterna, and right-sided termination. (From Davis, 1915.)

territories of the inferior mesenteric artery and the paired branches of the aorta, including the iliac arteries, plus two small azygos trunks which descend from the lower posterior intercostal regions. At its termination, the thoracic duct receives the left bronchomediastinal, internal jugular, and subclavian trunks.

On the right side the three trunks just named enter separately into the internal jugular or the subclavian vein. Uncommonly, they join to form a 'right lymph duct' prior to the venous termination.

VARIATIONS

A recognizable cisterna is formed in somewhat over half of all subjects; in the others, the trunks that usually enter

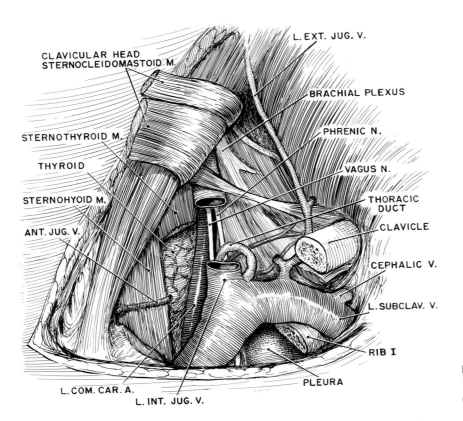

Labels on figure:
CLAVICULAR HEAD
STERNOCLEIDOMASTOID M.

L. EXT. JUG. V.

BRACHIAL PLEXUS

PHRENIC N.

STERNOTHYROID M.

THYROID

VAGUS N.

STERNOHYOID M.

THORACIC
DUCT

ANT. JUG. V.

CLAVICLE

CEPHALIC V.

L. SUBCLAV. V.

RIB I

L. COM. CAR. A.

PLEURA

L. INT. JUG. V.

FIG. 133
Termination of the thoracic duct.
(*After Cunningham, 1921.*)

a cisterna join in a plexus from which the thoracic duct arises
(Fig. 132). The upper boundary of the cisterna when formed
usually lies at the second lumbar vertebra, but may reach
as high as the twelfth thoracic.

Major variations of the thoracic duct itself include doubling, left sidedness, and right or bilateral termination, as
well as the very rare azygos vein termination (Fig. 132). The
embryologic basis for these variations is the plexiform nature
of the trunks from which the duct arises. Doubling is reported
in 4.7 per cent by Adachi (1953) and in 39 per cent in
a larger series by Van Pernis (1949): the lower figure is
probably correct for extensive duplication. In a few instances,
the abdominal components of the trunk may pass upward
to both sides or only to the left of the aorta. Rarely, the duct
may be left sided throughout its course (Adachi, 1953;
Davis, 1915). Only the upper part of the duct may be double
so that it terminates in both the right and left sides of the
neck (1.8 per cent) or the right side alone (1.6 per cent)
(Adachi, 1953). At its termination, the duct may enter into
a short plexus with its tributary trunks so that in about 20

per cent it enters the vein by two or more branches. Termination of the duct in the azygos system is quite rare. One of us (EAE), in an autopsy subject, has seen the duct enter the hemiazygos vein.

In its cervical course, the duct may run posterior rather than anterior to the vertebral or the subclavian artery (Adachi, 1953). Right-sided termination is said to be relatively common in cases of retro-esophageal right subclavian artery. In one case of situs inversus, Adachi found that the course of the duct was the mirror image of the usual. In three cases of aortic anomalies, there were other variations of position and termination.

COLLATERALS FOR THE THORACIC DUCT

Ligation of the thoracic duct is almost invariably adequately compensated for by collaterals. Ehrenhaft and Meyers (1948), for example, found that after an inadvertent ligation during a right supradiaphragmatic splanchnicectomy, the patient's blood fat content rose to normal levels in two weeks. The work of Lee (1922) in the dog suggests that collateral flow is either to a right duct or other lymphatic ducts or to a communication with the azygos system. Recent lymphangiographic studies indicate that lymphaticovenous communications may be widespread in man (Threefoot, 1968). Acute dilatation of the duct below a ligature has suggested to some (Hodge and Bridges, 1948; Brewer, 1955) the need to implant the distal segment into an adjacent vein (Fig. 134). The lower azygos vein lies beneath the right crus of the diaphragm adjacent to the duct; the hemiazygos generally pierces the left crus close to the aorta. Either vein, but especially the azygos, may be rudimentary in this region.

EXPOSURES OF THE THORACIC DUCT
AND CISTERNA CHYLI

Exposure of the cervical part of the thoracic duct is gained by dividing the clavicular origin of the sternocleidomastoid muscle, and searching in the jugular-subclavian venous angle for the thin-walled duct as it arches downward to its

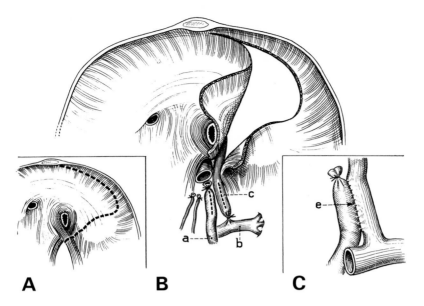

FIG. 134

Transsthoracic ligation of the cisterna chyli for left chylothorax, with decompressive lymphaticovenous anastomosis. A. The incision in the diaphragm. B. Ligation of the cisterna (a) and two lymph trunks. Ligation of the hemiazygos vein (c) at its junction with the left renal vein (b). C. Anastomosis (e) of the cisterna and hemiazygos vein. (From Carayon et al., 1963, after Brewer, 1955.)

termination (Figs. 132 and 133). The contents of the duct are yellow-white in color, the valves at its termination preventing a reflux of blood. If the duct is not seen at once, dissection should be carried medially beneath the internal jugular vein and carotid sheath. The vertebral vein lies immediately posterior to the internal jugular vein here (see Fig. 1). As noted, the duct may enter this vein or rarely run deep to it or the underlying artery (Tilney and Murray, 1968). The apical endothoracic fascia and the pleura lie beneath the duct proximal to its termination.

Within the thorax, the duct from T5 down is easily available after incising the right pleura anterior to the azygos vein. The duct has been injured here in performing splanchnicectomy, and Hodge and Bridges (1948) have implanted the duct into the azygos vein. Injuries on the left side have usually occurred during esophageal dissection in the apex of the thorax.

Intentional exposures of the thoracic portion of the duct have been few, except for simple ligation. The presence of a left chylothorax has led to left-sided approaches even for the lowest part of the duct. Thus, Lampson (1948) approached the duct through a left thoracotomy, dissecting anterior to the descending aorta. He showed a diagram of a similar approach posterior to the descending aorta used in a case by Meade. Such an anterior approach carries the hazard of division of nutrient arteries to the esophagus, and the posterior approach carries the hazard of division of an intercostal artery which may supply an important branch to the spinal cord (p. 73).

The cisterna chyli and thoracic duct have been exposed by Brewer (1955) (Fig. 134), by left thoracotomy and trans-diaphragmatic incision. On the right the liver prevents an ample opening of the diaphragm anterior to the duct and cisterna. Carayon *et al.* (1963) suggest an approach to the cisterna and duct by a left posterior retropleural and trans-diaphragmatic incision removing the twelfth rib. Their suggested method requires displacing the aorta forward to get across to the right side. If a posterior view sufficed, it would seem that a similar but right-sided approach would be more direct.

REFERENCES

Adachi, B.: Der Ductus thoracicus der Japaner. Tokyo, Kenkyusha, 1953.

Brewer, L. A., III: Surgical management of lesions of the thoracic duct. The technic and indications for retroperitoneal anastomosis of the thoracic duct to the hemiazygos vein. Amer. J. Surg. 90:210–227, 1955.

Carayon, A., Blanc, J.-F., and Bourrel, P.: Les ruptures du canal thoracique sous-diaphragmatique par contusions de l'abdomen. J. Chir. 86:177–190, 1963.

Davis, H. K.: A statistical study of the thoracic duct in man. Amer. J. Anat. 17:211–244, 1915.

Ehrenhaft, J. L., and Meyers, R.: Blood fat levels following supra-diaphragmatic ligation of the thoracic duct. Ann. Surg. 128:38–45, 1948.

Hodge, G. B., and Bridges, H.: Surgical management of thoracic duct injuries. An experimental study with clinical application. Surgery 24:805–810, 1948.

Lampson, R. S.: Traumatic chylothorax. A review of the literature and report of a case treated by mediastinal ligation of the thoracic duct. J. Thor. Surg. 17:778–791, 1948.

Lee, F. C.: The establishment of collateral circulation following ligation of the thoracic duct. Bull. Johns Hopkins Hosp. 33:21–31, 1922.

Threefoot, S. A.: Lymphaticovenous communications. Chapter II *in* Lymph and the Lymphatic System. Proceedings of the Conference on Lymph and the Lymphatic System, Mayerson, H. S., Chairman. Springfield, Charles C Thomas, 1968.

Tilney, N. L., and Murray, J. E.: Chronic thoracic duct fistula. Operative technic and physiologic effects in man. Ann. Surg. 167:1–8, 1968.

Van Pernis, P. A.: Variations of the thoracic duct. Surgery 26:806–809, 1949.

iNdEx

Page numbers in *italics* refer to illustrations.

ABBOTT'S ARTERY, 59, *61*
Abdominal disease, scalene-node biopsy in, 33
Abdominal ganglion removal, 24
Abscess, hepatic or subhepatic, 199
    transpleural approach to, *205*
    pulmonary, 171
Accessory nerve, 10, *12*
Adenomas, parathyroid, intrathoracic, 83, *84*
Adrenal gland, biopsy of, 21, *23*
    denervation of, 20
    exposure of, 21, *23*, 24
    left, 205
    right, 199
Air embolism, 34
Alveolar pores, 170
Amputation, interscapulothoracic, 10
    exposure for, *11*
Aneurysm, aortic, exposure for, 45
    paraplegia following, 74, 75
    ventricular, 210
Angina pectoris, neurectomy for, 149, *154*, 157
    sympathectomy for, 156
Ansa subclavia, 97
    damage to, 45
Anuli, cardiac, *103*, 104, 135
Aorta, anomalies of, 53–56, *55*, 177
    ascending, mid-sternal approach to, 44
        in cardiac transplantation, 138, *139*
    bronchial branches of, 64, 66, *69*
    coarctation of, 45, 58–61
        collateral circulation in, *59*
        exposures for, *60, 61*
        paraplegia following, 74
    descending, 29, 64, *65*
        exposure of, 45
    descending thoracic, 63, 64
    dextroposition of, 124
    esophageal branches of, 71
    exposures of, 44–52
        lymphatics and, *160*
    in double-outlet right ventricle, 110
    in thoracic duct surgery, 233
    intercostal branches of, 64
    paraplegia and, 74, 75
    proximal, 98
    right dorsal, 64
    wall of, *105*
Aortic anulus, *103*
Aortic arch, 29
    branches of, normal variations in, 40–43, *41*
    double, 53, *55*, 56, 57
    embryonic, 53, *54*
    exposure of, 44, 45

    in intrathoracic goiter, 79
    in mediastinoscopy, 35, 38
    in tracheal surgery, 192
    inferior laryngeal nerve and, 81
    receptor areas in, 156
    right, 56
        doubling of vena cava and, 112
        left ductus and, 57
    thyroidea ima arterial branch of, *81*
Aortic insufficiency, 111
Aortic stenosis, calcific, 110
Aortic valve, 108–114
    blood supply to, 144, 145
    circumference of, 105, *106*
    distortion of, 105
    exposure of, *109*, 110–111
    replacement of, 105
        atrioventricular bundle in, 103, 111
            injury to, 135
        mitral insufficiency and, 110
Aortography, paraplegia following, 76
Aorto-pulmonary anastomosis, 188
Aperture, superior thoracic, 3–9
Apicolysis, extrafascial, 6, 13–14, *14*
Apicoposterior trunk, 187, *188*
Arcuate ligaments, 208, *209*
    in hiatus hernia repair, *215*, 216
Arm, Blalock operation and, 45
    denervation of, 16
    pedicle exposure of, 10
Arteria aberrans, 54, *65*
Arteria radicularis magna, 74
Arteriography, paraplegia following, 75
Artery(ies). See names of specific arteries.
Aspiration, of foreign material, 171
    pericardial, 162–164, *163*
Atrial appendage, 97, 102
Atrial internodal conduction tracts, 132, *133*, 134
Atrial septum, 115
    defects of. See *Interatrial septal defects.*
    embryology of, 119, *120*
    in cardiac transplantation, 138
Atrioventricular block, 117
Atrioventricular bundle, 103, 132, *133*
    course of, 134, 135
    in aortic valve replacement, 103, 111, 135
    innervation of, 156
    right branch of, 118
    suture of, 136
Atrioventricular canal, endocardial cushions of, 119
    defects of, 115
Atrioventricular conduction, aberrant, 136
    surgery and, 124

Atrioventricular groove, 97, 108
    dehiscence of, 104
    in pericardiectomy, 164
Atrioventricular node, 117, 132, *133, 134*
    bypass of, 136
    in atrial septal defect, *133,* 134
    injury to, 135
    innervation of, 156
Atrioventricular node artery, *104,* 145, 146
    anomalous origin of, *143,* 144, 146
Atrioventricular orifice, abnormality of, 129
Atrioventricular perimeter, 103–106, *104*
Atrioventricular valves, 118
    anulus of, 104
    dysfunction of, 160
    rings of, 103
Atrium(a), approach to, right-sided, 100–107, *101*
    blood supply to, 69, 144–147
    embryonic, 117
    in cardiac transplantation, 138, 146
        Shumway technique for, *139,* 157
    innervation of, 156
    left, *187*
        enlargement of, 172
        in pneumonectomy, 184
            incision of, *101,* 102, 108, *109*
            interior of, 108–110, *109*
            superior vena cava opening into, 112
        oblique ligament of, 111, 156
    myocardium of, 134
    right, 97, 115–123
        networks in, 119–122, *121*
        in mitral valve replacement, 102
        incision of, 134
        interior of, 115–118, *116*
        valves of, 119–122, *120, 121*
Auricular anastomotic artery, *104, 142,* 144, 145
    communication with atrioventricular node artery, 146
Axilla, cervicothoracic sympathectomy through, 16
    exposure for, 49, *51*
    rib removal through, 6, *7*
Axillary veins, 49
    exposure of, 50
Azygos lobe, 167, *169*
Azygos lymph node, 182
Azygos vein, 72, *187*
    arch of, 29
    in cardiac surgery, 100, *101*
    in esophagectomy, 223, 225, 226
    in intrathoracic goiter, 79, 80
    in mediastinoscopy, 38
    in pneumonectomy, 183
    in superior vena cava anomaly, 112
    in tracheal exposure, 192
    thoracic duct implantation into, 232
    thoracic duct termination in, *229,* 230, 231

BACHMANN'S BUNDLE, 134
Balloon catheter, intravascular, 50
Baroreceptors, atrial, 139
Biopsy, mediastinal, *37*
    of adrenal gland, 21, *23*
    of internal thoracic lymph nodes, 15
    of kidney, 21, *23*
    of lung tissue, 33
    of parasternal lymph nodes, 33
    of pretracheal and paratracheal lymph nodes, 35, 36
    of scalene fat, 35

of scalene lymph nodes, 33, 183
of superior sulcus tumor, 34
of tracheobronchial lymph nodes, 36
Blalock subclavian–pulmonary artery anastomosis, 44, 45, *46*
Bleeding, mediastinoscopy-induced, 38
Blood samples, cardiac, 117
Bochdalek's foramen, 209
    hernia of, 178
Boyd's repair of hiatus hernia, 206, *215*
Brachial plexus, 3, *4*
    exposure of, 50
    in rib removal, 6, *7*
    in sternotomy, 95
    in thoracoplasty, 13
    origin of, *17*
    root injury to, 12
Brachiocephalic trunk, 193
    anomalous, 56, 63
        approach to, 57
    coronary system originating from, 127
    exposure for, 44
    suspension of, 56, 57
    thyroidea ima artery arising from, *80,* 81
    variations in, 40, *41*
Brachiocephalic vein(s), 48
    exposure of, 50
    in mediastinoscopy, 38
    in vascular ring surgery, 57
    injury to, 35
    left, 86, 95, *155*
        in tracheal exposure, 193
        retro-aortic, 111–114, *113*
        small, 98, 112
    right, 111
Brain, blood supply to, 63
Breast, blood supply of, 64, 65
    surgery of, *14, 15*
        approach for, 33
Bronchial arterial tree occlusion, 70
Bronchial arteriography, paraplegia following, 75
Bronchial artery(ies), 63, 65–70, 176
    cervical tracheo-esophageal artery anastomosis with, 71
    coronary artery anastomosis with, 146
    division of, 59, 147
    esophageal branches of, 71, 224
    in pulmonary embolism, 72
    in pulmonary resection, 180
    left view of, *68*
    pulmonary artery anastomosis with, *70*
    right, anomalous, *69*
    right view of, *67*
    sinu-atrial branch of, *145,* 147
Bronchial veins, 72, 176
    in pulmonary embolism, 72
Bronchomediastinal lymph trunk, 182, 229
Bronchoscopy, 170–172, *171*
Bronchus(i), atrial enlargement and, 172
    blood supply of, 63, 64
    branching of, *176, 177*
    bronchoscopic view of, 170–172, *171*
    compression of, 56
    eparterial, 171, 176
    in tracheal resection, 193, *194*
    left, 188, *189*
    occlusion of, 169
    right, *185–187*
        exposure of, 192
    variations of, 177
Bulbospiral muscles, *119*

Burns' suprasternal space, 93
Bursa, infracardiac, *211*
    omental, 205
Bypass grafting of esophagus, 219

CALCIFICATION OF CARDIAC SYSTEM, 110, 135
Canal of Søndergaard, *101, 102*
Cancer, esophageal, 218, 219, 223
    pulmonary, 33, 70
    thyroidal, 78, *79*
    tracheal, 195
Capitis muscle, 42
Cardia of stomach, esophageal carcinoma and, 218
Cardiac. See also *Heart.*
Cardiac catheterization, 117
Cardiac conduction system, 132–137, *133*
    surgery and, 124
Cardiac ganglion, 153, *155*
Cardiac lymphatics, 159–161, *160*
    in transplantation, 138, 139, 160
    injury to, 98
Cardiac nerves, 153–158, *154, 155*
    in transplantation, 138, 139, 157
    injury to, 98
Cardiac pain, neurectomy for, 157
    sensation of, 153, 154
    sympathectomy for, 156
        approach to, 157
Cardiac plexus(es), 153, 154, *155*
    distribution from, 156
    in cardiac transplantation, 157
Cardiac revascularization, 141–152
Cardiac skeleton, 103–106, *103*
Cardiac surgery, catheterization during, 110, 126
    vena cava in, *101, 102,* 112
Cardiac transplantation, 138–140, *139*
    collateral circulation following, 146
    innervation in, 138, 139, 157
    lymphatics in, 138, 139, 160
Cardiac valves. See specific valves.
Cardiac veins, *104,* 147, *148,* 149
Cardio-esophageal angulation, 211
Cardiopulmonary bypass, 117
    in heart transplantation, 138, *139*
Carina, tracheal, in bronchoscopy, 170
    nodes of, 36
Carotid artery(ies), common, anomalous, 40, 42, *83*
    cervical tracheo-esophageal branch of, 71
    left, anomalous, 40, *41*
        approaches to, 44, 57
        suspension of, *56*
    right, anomalous, 40, *41*
        thyroidea ima artery arising from, 81
        vertebral arterial branch of, 82, *83*
    exposure of, 50
    internal, 63
        anomalous, *41*
            right vertebral arterial branch of, 42
Carotid sheath, exposure of, 47
    in mediastinoscopy, 35
Cartilage. See also names of specific cartilages.
    healing of, 222, 225
Catheter, balloon, intravascular, 50
    pacemaker, 118
Catheterization, coronary artery variations and, 126, 127
    for cardiopulmonary bypass, 117
    for ventricular decompression, 110

Caval cardiac node, 159
Celiac ganglion removal, 24
Cephalic vein, 49
Cervical artery(ies), 17
    transverse, *12,* 17
        branches of, 10, 12, 58
Cervical esophagus, blood supply of, 64
Cervical ganglion, *155*
    fusion with thoracic nerve, 16
    vascular deprivation of, 45
Cervical nerve, eighth, 3, *5*
    root injury to, 12
Cervical rib removal, *7*
    approaches to, 8
Cervical spinal cord, blood supply of, 64
Cervical thyroid, 79
Cervical tracheo-esophageal arteries, 71, 192, *193*
Cervical vein, deep, 48
Cervical vertebra, 42
Cervico-axillary extensions of sternotomy, 49–51
Cervicodorsal sympathectomy, 156
    approach to, 157
Cervicomediastinal exploration, 35
    complications in, 38
    suprasternal approach to, *36, 37*
Cervicothoracic exposure, by sternoclavicular elevation,
        49
    by sternoclaviculopectoral pedicle, 49, *50*
    of thyroid, parathyroids, or thymus, 47
Cervicothoracic ganglion, 3, *4, 5, 155*
    in cervicothoracic sympathectomy, 16, *17*
        exposure of, 18, *19*
    removal of, 7
        for cardiac pain, 156
Cervicothoracic-axillary exposure, 49, *51*
Chiari network, *121, 122*
Chordae tendineae, 110, 117
Chylothorax, *232*
Circumflex coronary arteries, *104,* 110, 141, *143*
    atrioventricular node artery arising from, 146
    catheterization of, 127
    in mitral valve replacement, 105
    origin from right coronary artery, 127, *128*
Cisterna chyli, 228, 230
    absence of, *229*
    exposures for, 231–233, *232*
Clavicle, excision of, 48
    in cervicothoracic-axillary exposure, 49, *51*
Claviculopectoral pedicle, 49
Clavipectoral fascia, *8*
    in rib removal, 6
Coarctation of aorta. See *Aorta, coarctation of.*
Collar incision, 47
    for thymus exposure, 87
    for thyroidectomy, *79*
    for tracheal resection, 195
Colon, esophageal replacement with, 220, *222*
    hepatic flexure of, 199
    splenic flexure of, 205
Commissures of heart, 117
Congenital heart disease, 110, 124–131. See also specific
        diseases.
    anomalous coronary arteries in, 127
    cyanotic, 95
    surgery for, atrioventricular block following, 117
        conduction injury during, 132
    tracheal compression in, 57
Conus ligament, *103*
Conus of right ventricle, 118

Coronary artery(ies), 141–152
    anomalies of, 124, 126–130, *126, 128, 129*
    circumflex, *104,* 110, 141, *143*
        atrioventricular node artery arising from, 146
        catheterization of, 127
        in mitral valve replacement, 105
        origin from right coronary artery, 127, *128*
    collaterals for, 146–147
    conus, 97, 124
        separate, 126
    diameters of, 149
    distribution patterns of, 141–144, *142, 143*
    occlusion of, 141, 146
    reconstruction of, 149
    right, 97, *104*
        distal, 110
        lymphatics and, 159
    single, *126*
    sinu-atrial artery arising from, 144
Coronary artery disease, 110
Coronary plexuses, 153, 156
Coronary system, external collaterals for, 147
    extracoronary artery communications of, 149
Coronary tree, 64
Coronary vein(s), 72, 141–152
    great, 147, *148*
        ligation of, 149
Coronary venous sinus, *104,* 147–149, *148*
    in left cardiac exposures, 111
    mediastinal veins and, communication of, 146
    orifice of, 115, *116*
        atresia of, 112
    valves of, 119, *120*
        fenestrations of, 122
Costal cartilage, in esophagectomy, 225
    in mediastinal biopsy, *37*
    in sympathectomy, 16
    removal of, 12, 33, *37*
    sectioning of, 48
Costocervical trunk, 3, *4, 5*
    anomalous, 42, *43*
    branches of, bronchial arterial, 66
        superior intercostal, 64
    connection to descending aorta, 64, *65*
    in Blalock operation, 45
Costo-coracoid fascia, 49
Costophrenic sinuses, 199
    obliteration of, *205*
Costotransverse ligament, *13*
Costovertebral junctions, *13*
Costovertebral ligament, *13*
Costovertebral trunk, 74
Crista supraventricularis, 118, 124
Crista terminalis, *116,* 117
    embryology of, 119
Crura of diaphragm, 208, *209*
    esophageal hiatus and, 211, *215*
    in esophageal surgery, 225
    in hiatus hernia repair, *215,* 216
    vasculature of, 207
Cushion, endocardial, congenital defects of, 115
    embryology of, 119
Cyanotic congenital heart disease, 95
Cysts, mediastinoscopic emptying of, 38

Deltopectoral triangle, 49
Dextrocardia, 157

Diaphragm, 199, *209*
    crura of, 208, *209*
        esophageal hiatus and, 211, *215*
        in esophageal surgery, 225
        in hiatus hernia repair, *215,* 216
        vasculature of, 207
    in esophageal surgery, 222
    in median sternotomy, 93, *94*
    phrenic nerve branching on, *206*
Diaphragmatic hernia, 178, 208–210, *210*
Double-outlet right ventricle, 110
Ductus arteriosus, 53, *55,* 82
    division of, 56
    in coarctation surgery, 58
    lymph nodes of, 182
    patent, 57–58
        exposure for, *58*
        left superior vena cava and, 112
Duval-Barasty exposure, 93

Embolism, air, 34
    paradoxical, 122
    pulmonary artery, 72, 180
Embryo, aortic arches of, 53, *54*
    heart of, 119, *120*
Endarterectomy, coronary artery, 149
Endo-abdominal fascia, 212
Endocardial cushions, defects of, 115
    embryology of, 119
Endocardial fibrosis, 160
Endocardium, 115
Endometriosis, diaphragmatic perforation by, 210
Endothoracic fascia, 4, 6. See also *Suprapleural membrane.*
    in cervicothoracic sympathectomy, 16
Endotracheal tubes, tracheal injuries due to, 192
Eparterial bronchus, 171, 176
Epicardium in mitral valve replacement, 102
Erector spinae muscles, in cervicothoracic sympathectomy, 18
    in thoracoplasty, 12
Esophageal artery(ies), *67, 68,* 70–72
    bronchial vessels from, 69
    division of, 59, 233
    in esophagectomy, 224
    intercostal arterial sources of, 65, *66,* 71
Esophageal atresia, extrapleural approach to, *225, 226*
Esophageal bypass, 219, *220, 221*
Esophageal hiatus, *209*
    hernia of, 210–216
        operations for, 206, *215,* 216
        stomach in, 212, *213*
        thoracic approach to, *214,* 215
        varieties of, *213*
    origin of, 211
Esophageal varices, 72
Esophageal veins, 72, *73*
Esophagectomy, approaches for, 206
    high thoracic, 225–226
    low thoracic, 222–224, *223*
Esophagogastric junction, *211,* 212
    in hiatus hernia repair, *214*
Esophagogastric resection, 72
Esophagogastrostomy, 222–224, *223, 224*
    approaches for, 206
Esophago-ileocolic-gastrostomy, 220, *221*
Esophagus, 29, *187*
    approaches to, extrapleural, 6, 33, *225, 226*
        right-sided, 225–226

Esophagus (*Continued*)
    arteries to, 64, 70–72, 81
    cancer of, 218, 219, 223
    compression of, 56
    course of, 218
    dissection of, 232
    divisions of, physiologic, 70, *211*
    in mediastinoscopy, 38
    resection and replacement of, 218–227, *221, 222*
        high thoracic, 72
        structures for, 219–222
    sphincter of, *211, 212*
    thoracic, blood supply to, 69
    vagal branches to, 188
    venous drainage of, 72, *73*
Eustachian ridge, 134
Eustachian valve, 117
Extrafascial apicolysis, 6, 13–14, *14*
Extralobar sequestration, 178
    hernia complicating, 209
Extraperitoneal approach to subphrenic and subhepatic
        spaces, *205*
Extrapleural approach, cleavage plane in, 6
    to anterolateral thoracotomy, 44
    to ductus arteriosus, 57
    to esophagus, *225,* 226
    to subclavian artery, 45, *47*
    to sympathectomy, 10, *20,* 33
        to cervicothoracic, 18
    to thymus, 87
Extrapleural drainage of mediastinum, 6
    by mediastinotomy, 33, *34, 35*
Extremity, upper, Blalock operation and, 45
    denervation of, 16
    pedicle exposure of, 10

FALLOT'S TETRALOGY. See *Tetralogy of Fallot.*
Fascia(e). See names of specific fasciae.
Fat, preperitoneal, 93
    scalene, biopsy of, 35
Fat pads, scalene and prescalene, 33
Fibrosis, of endocardium, 160
    of papillary muscle, 110
Fibrous anuli of heart, *103,* 135
    fila coronaria in, *103,* 104
Fibrous anuli of heart, *103,* 115
Fibrous trigones of heart, *103,* 115
Fila coronaria, *103,* 104
Fistula, lymph, 34
Foramen, transverse, vertebral artery entering, 42
Foramen magnum, 48
Foramen of Bochdalek, 209
    hernia of, 178
Foramen of Morgagni, hernia of, 209, *210*
Foramen ovale, 119
    patent, *121,* 122
Foramen primum defect, 119
    atrioventricular node artery in, 146
    atrioventricular node in, *133,* 134
    closure of, 135
Foramen secundum defect, 122, *125,* 126
    embryology of, 119
Fossa ovalis, 115
    limbus of, *116,* 117
    sinus venosus network in, 117, 119, *120, 121,* 122

GANGLION(A). See names of specific ganglia.
Gangrene of arm, 45

Gastrectomy, 72, 219
Gastric artery(ies), 63, 71
    in esophageal surgery, 219
Gastric lymph nodes, 219
Gastric vein, left, 72
Gastroepiploic artery, 219
Goiter, 78–80
Grafting, for esophageal replacement, 219, *222*
    for myocardial revascularization, 149
    for tracheal reconstruction, 195
Great vessels, 29, 48
    abnormalities of, 53–62. See also specific abnormalities.
    approaches to, 6, 44–52, *47,* 93
    in mediastinoscopy, 38
    pericardial attachment to, 100–102
    vasa vasorum of, 98, 146

HEART, 29, 93–164. See also *Cardiac* and specific
        structures.
    approaches to, 100, 108, *109*
    blood samples from, 117
    coronary arteries communicating with, 127, *129*
    embryology of, 119, *120*
    injured in pericardiectomy, 164
    junctional zone of, 141
    pressure reception in, 153, 156
    revascularization of, 141–152
    sensory denervation of, 16
    skeleton of, 103–106, *103*
    views of, 95–98
Heart block, surgical production of, 136
Heart disease, congenital. See *Congenital heart disease* and
        specific diseases.
Hemiazygos vein, 72, *73*
    thoracic duct implantation in, 231, *232*
Hemorrhage, mediastinoscopy-induced, 38
Hemothorax, 210
Hepatic abscess, 199
    transpleural approach to, *205*
Hepatic artery, esophageal branches of, 71
Hepatic flexure, 199
Hernia, diaphragmatic, 178, 208–210, *210*
    hiatus, 210–216
        operations for, 206, *215,* 216
        stomach in, 212, *213*
        thoracic approach to, *214,* 215
        varieties of, *213*
Hiatus, esophageal, *209*
    origin of, 211
Horizontal fissure of lung, 167
Horner's syndrome, 16
    Blalock's operation and, 45
    mediastinotomy and, 34
Hypertension, pulmonary venous, 108
    sympathectomy for, 20
Hypoglossal canal, 42

ILIAC ARTERY, in coarctation of aorta, *59*
Infarction of papillary muscle, 110
Infracardiac bursa, *211*
Infrahyoid fascia, 36, 48
    in cervico-axillary extension of sternotomy, 50
    in thymus surgery, 87
Infrahyoid muscles, 36, 48
    in cervico-axillary extension of sternotomy, 50
    in thymus surgery, 87
Infundibulum, right ventricular, 118

Innominate artery. See *Brachiocephalic trunk.*
Insufflation, intratracheal, 169
Interalveolar openings, 170
Interatrial foramen I defect, 119
　atrioventricular node artery in, 146
　atrioventricular node in, *133,* 134
　closure of, 135
Interatrial foramen II defect, 122, *125,* 126
　embryology of, 119, *120*
Interatrial groove, *101,* 102
　surgical procedures and, 145
Interatrial septal defects, 122
　canal of Søndergaard in, 102
　coronary variations and, 129
　primum type of, 119
　　atrioventricular node in, *133,* 134
　　atrioventricular node artery in, 146
　　closure of, 135
　secundum type of, 122, *125,* 126
　　embryology of, 119, *120*
　　vena caval anomaly and, 112
Interatrial septum(a), 115
　embryology of, 119, *120*
　in cardiac transplantation, 138
Interclavicular ligament, 93
Intercostal artery(ies), 63, 64-65, *65*
　anomalous, *94,* 95
　aortic, 74
　bronchial branches of, 66, 68, *69, 70*
　esophageal branches of, 65, *66,* 71
　highest, 17
　in coarctation surgery, 59, *60*
　in thoracic duct surgery, 233
　in Vineberg procedure, 150
　radicular branches of, 74
　visceral branches of, 65, *66*
Intercostal bundles, division of, 58
Intercostal muscles, 57, 58
Intercostal nerves, *13,* 64
　ablation of, 18
　exposure of, 19
　in cardiac innervation, 153, 154
Intercostal vessels, *13,* 111
　in esophageal surgery, 223
Interlobar vein, 167
Internodal tracts, 132, *133,* 134
Interscapulothoracic amputation, 10
　exposure for, *11*
Intersegmental veins, 170
Interventricular artery, anterior, anomalous, 97
　　great cardiac vein and, 149
　　in parasternal puncture, *163,* 164
　　in tetralogy of Fallot surgery, 129
　　intramural, *126,* 127
　　origin from right coronary artery, 124, 127, *128*
　left anterior, 110
　posterior, in unbalanced circulation, 141, *142, 143*
Interventricular septal defect, 124, *125*
　conduction elements and, *133*
　coronary artery variations and, 129
　repair of, 135
Interventricular septum, *105*
　as junctional zone, 141
Intervertebral foramina, 64
Intestinal lymph trunk, 228
Intestine for esophageal bypass, 219, *220, 221*
Intracranial arteries, 63, 74
Intralobar sequestration, 178
Intratracheal goiter, 80

Intratracheal insufflation, 169
Intravertebral plexus, 48

JACKSON-HUBER SYSTEM OF CLASSIFICATION, *168,* 170, *171*
Jejunum for esophageal bypass, 219, *220,* 221
Jugular arch, anterior, 36
Jugular lymphatics, 33, 182, 229
　metastasis to, 183
Jugular veins, 111, 182, 229
　in cervico-axillary extension of sternotomy, 50
　in cervicothoracic sympathectomy, 16, *19*
　in median sternotomy, 93
　in mediastinoscopy, 35
　in mediastinotomy, 34
　injury to, 48
　posterior, 48
Junctional zone, of heart, 141
　of spinal cord, 74
Juxta-esophageal nodes, 222

KIDNEY, 209
　exposure of, 21, *23,* 24
　upper poles of, 199, 205
Kocher maneuver, 219
Kohn's alveolar pores, 170
Kugel's artery, *104, 142,* 144, 145
　atrioventricular node artery communication with, 146

LARYNGEAL NERVE(S), inferior, 81-83, *82, 84*
　recurrent, 83, *155,* 156, 173
　　in coarctation surgery, 58
　　in mediastinoscopy, 38
　　in patent ductus arteriosus, 57, *58*
　　in subclavian artery surgery, 57
　　left, 224
Larynx, blood supply of, 64
Latissimus dorsi muscle, in coarctation surgery, 58
　in thoracoplasty, 10
Levator scapulae muscle, 10, *12*
Ligamentum arteriosum, 173, 188
　origin of, 156
　recurrent laryngeal nerve and, 83
Linea alba in median sternotomy, 93
Lingula of lung, 167, *168*
Lingular artery, *188*
Lingular bronchi, 172
Lingular vein, *188*
Lingulectomy, *190,* 191
Linton's sympathectomy, *22,* 206
Liver, 199
　abscess of, 199
　　transpleural approach to, *205*
　in hiatus hernia repair, 216
Longus colli muscle, 42
Limbus of fossa ovalis, *116,* 117
Lumbar arteries, 74
Lumbar lymph trunks, 228
Lumbocostal arches, 208, *209*
　in hiatus hernia repair, *215,* 216
Lungs, 167-196. See also *Pulmonary.*
　abscesses of, 171
　aspiration of foreign material into, 171
　biopsy of, 33
　bronchovascular distribution in, 169
　cancer of, 33, 70
　collapse of, surgical, 6, 13-14, *14*

Lungs (*Continued*)
  fissures of, 167–168, *168*
  for coronary–extracoronary artery communication, 149
  hila of, anatomy of, 184–191
    blood supply to, 69
    dissection of, 184, *185*, 188
    exposure of, 44
    in mediastinoscopy, 38
    view of, 185, *186, 187, 188, 189*
    in tracheal resection, 193, 194
  left, branching of bronchi and blood vessels in, *177*
    surgery of, 112
  lingula of, 167, *168*
  lobes of, 167–168, *168, 169*
  osteoarthropathy of, 38
  resection of, 173, 184–191
    bronchial arteries in, 180
  right, blood supply to, 65, *67*
    branching of bronchi and blood vessels in, *176*
  root of, 29, 173–180
    left view of, *31, 175*
    right view of, *30, 174*
  segments of, *168,* 169–170
Lymph fistula, 34
Lymphaticovenous anastomosis, *232*
Lymphatic nodes and vessels, bronchomediastinal, 182, 229
  cardiac, 159–161, *160*
    in transplantation, 138, 139, 160
    injury to, 98
  gastric, 219
  in esophageal surgery, 219, 222
  in pulmonary ligament, 182
    removal of, 219
  internal thoracic, biopsy of, 15
  jugular, 33, 182, 229
    metastasis to, 183
  juxta-esophageal, 222
  lumbar, 228
  mediastinal, 159
    removal in esophageal surgery, 219
  para-aortic, 228
  parasternal, 159
    biopsy of, 33
  paratracheal, *181*
    biopsy of, 35, 36
  pretracheal, biopsy of, 35, 36
  pulmonary, 176, 180–183, *187*
    anterior and posterior views of, *181*
    overall view of, *180*
  scalene, 33, 182, 229
    biopsy of, 33, 183
  subclavian, 182, 229
  thoracic, in extrafascial apicolysis, *14*
    internal, biopsy of, 15
    removal of, *15*
  tracheobronchial, 36, 159, *181*
    exposure of, 33

Mammalian embryo, aortic arches of, 53, *54*
  heart of, 119, *120*
Mammary artery(ies). See *Thoracic artery(ies), internal.*
Mammectomy, *14, 15*
  approach for, 33
Manubrium, in cervicothoracic exposure, 49
  in median sternotomy, 95
Marshall's ligament, 111, 156
Marshall's oblique vein, 111, *148*

Mastectomy, *14, 15*
  approach for, 33
Mediastinal artery, 65, *66*
Mediastinal lymph nodes, 159
  removal in esophageal cancer surgery, 219
Mediastinal pleura, blood supply to, 64
Mediastinal veins, communication with coronary venous sinus, 146
Mediastinal viscera, blood supply of, 63
Mediastinitis, 33
Mediastinoscopy, 33–38, *36, 37*
  in thymus surgery, 87
Mediastinotomy, 33–38
  cervical, 33, *34*
  mid-sternal, 33, *94*
  posterior, *35*
    for esophagectomy, 226
    for thymus exposure, 87
Mediastinum, 29–39
  biopsy of, *37*
  blood supply to, 69
  boundaries and contents of, 29–32, *30–32*
  dissection of, 57
  esophageal veins in, 72
  extrapleural drainage of, 6
    by mediastinotomy, 33, *34, 35*
  goiter in, 78, 79
  great vessels of, approach to, 44, 93
  mid-sternal approach to, 33, *94*
  parathyroid tumors in, 83, *84*
  view of, *174, 175*
Metastases, to jugular lymphatics, 183
  to scalene lymph node, 183
  to thoracic duct, 33
Mid-sternal approach, to aorta and great vessels, 44
  to thymus, 87
Mitral "curtain," 108, *109*
Mital insufficiency, 110
Mitral stenosis, 110
Mitral valve, circumference of, 105, *106*
  cusps of, *105,* 108, 115, *116*
    accessory, 102
    injury to, 110
  distortion of, 105
  exposure of, from left, 108–114, *109*
    right atrial approach to, 134
  fila coronaria of, *103,* 104
  replacement of, 102–107, *101*
Moderator band, 118
  atrioventricular bundle branch in, 135
Morgagni's foramen, herniation through, 209, *210*
Muscle. See names of specific muscles.
Myocardial bundles, 124
Myocardium, atrial, 134
  interventricular arteries in, 127
  revascularization of, 149–151, *150*
  ventricular, 110
Myofibril network of Purkinje, 132, 136

Neck, esophageal veins in, 72
  exposure extended to, 47–48
  thymus in, 85
  vertebral arteries in, 74
Neoplasms. See *Tumors.*
Nephrectomy, 206
Nerve. See names of specific nerves.
Neurectomy for angina pectoris, 149, *154,* 157
Neurofibromas, paravertebral, 38

Neurovascular compression, exploration for, 17
  rib removal for, 6–8, *7*
    posterolateral approach to, 10
Newborn, thymus in, *85*

Oblique fissures of lung, 167, *168*
Oblique ligament of atrium, 111, 156
Oblique vein, 111, 147, *148*
Omentum, for coronary–extracoronary artery
    communication, 149
  lesser, 199
Omohyoid muscle, *155*
  in cervicothoracic sympathectomy, *18*
  in mediastinotomy, 34
Open heart surgery, catheterization during, 110, 126
  superior vena cava and, 112
Osteoarthropathy, pulmonary, 38

Pacemaker catheter, 118
Pain, cardiac, neurectomy for, 157
    sensation of, 153, 154
    sympathectomy for, 156
      approach to, 157
Papillary muscles, 110, *116*, 117
Para-aortic lymph trunks, 228
Paradoxical embolism, 122
Paraduodenal peritoneum in esophageal surgery, 219
Para-esophageal hernia, 212, *213*
  repair of, 216
Paraplegia, post-surgical, 74, 75, 76
Parascapular approach to rib, 8
Parascapular muscles, *11*
Parascapular structures, *12*
Parasternal lymph nodes, 159
  biopsy of, 33
Parasternal puncture, 162, *163*, 164
Parasympathetic innervation of heart, 153, 156
Parathyroid adenomas, intrathoracic, 83, *84*
Parathyroid glands, 78–89
  blood supply of, 64, 81
  exposure of, 47
  thymic rests of, 85, *86*
  tumors of, 83–84, *84*
Paratracheal lymph nodes, *181*
  biopsy of, 35, 36
Paravertebral neurofibromas, 38
Parenchyma, lung, blood supply to, 69
Parietal pleura in cervicothoracic sympathectomy,
  16
Pars bifurcalis, 71
Patent ductus arteriosus, 57–58
  exposure for, *58*
  left superior vena cava and, 112
Pectinate muscles, 117
Pectoralis major muscle, 15
  in cervicothoracic exposure, 49
  in median sternotomy, 93
  in rib removal, 8
Pectoralis minor muscle in rib removal, 6, *7*
'Pencil patency' of foramen ovale, 122
Peptic ulcer, 216
Pericardiacophrenic artery(ies), 64
  in mitral valve exposure, 108, *109*
  superior phrenic branches of, 207
Pericardiacophrenic veins, 108, *109*
Pericardiacosternal ligaments, 95

Pericardial arteries, *98*, 146
Pericardial attachment to great veins, 100–102
Pericardiectomy, *163*, 164
Pericardiocentesis and drainage, 162–164, *163*
Pericarditis, constrictive, 164
Pericardium, 90–164
  adhesions of, 149
  bare area of, 95, *96*
  blood supply to, 64, 69
  congenital defects of, 97
  cul-de-sac of, 100
  drainage of, 162, *163*
  in hiatus hernia repair, 215
  in mitral valve exposure, 108, *109*
  in tracheal resection, 194
  reflection of, lines of, 97, *98*
Pericoronary neurectomy, 149, 157
Periosteum, in apicolysis, 13
  in heart disease, 95
Peritoneal ligaments, in esophageal surgery, 219
Peritoneal relationships, subphrenic, *204*
Peritoneum, 199
  in esophageal surgery, 219
Pharyngeal arteries, 71
Pharynx, blood supply of, 64
Phrenic artery, inferior, 63, 207
  esophageal branches of, 71
Phrenic nerve, 17, 34, 48
  branching of, *206*
  in cardiac innervation, *155*
  in cervico-axillary extension of sternotomy, 50
  in cervicothoracic sympathectomy, *19*
  in esophageal surgery, 222
  in mitral valve exposure, 108, *109*
  in pulmonary resection, 187, *188*
  in rib removal, 7
  injury to, 206–207
    mediastinoscopy-induced, 38
Phreno-esophageal fascia, 212, *213*
  in hiatus hernia repair, *214*, 215
Pleura, 95
  apical structures of, *5*
  blood supply to, 64, 65
  in cervicothoracic sympathectomy, 16, 19
  in esophageal surgery, 223
  in hiatus hernia repair, 215
  in mastectomy, *14*, *15*
  in mediastinoscopy, 35
  in pneumonectomy, 183
  in thoracic duct exposures, 232
  in vascular ring surgery, 57
  reflection of, 95, *96*
Pleural sinuses, costophrenic, 199
Pleuroperitoneal canal, 209
Pneumonectomy, 6, 173
  in bronchial arterial tree occlusion, 70
  radical, 183–184
    left, *184*
    right, *182*, *183*
Pneumothorax, 15
  extrapleural, 6
  following parasternal puncture, 162
  mediastinoscopy-induced, 38
Portal obstruction, esophageal varices in, 72
Portapulmonary venous shunting, 73
Preperitoneal fat in median sternotomy, 93
Prescalene fat pad, 33
Pressure reception, cardiac, 153, 156
Pretracheal lymph node biopsy, 35, 36

'Probe patency' of foramen ovale, 122
Psoas muscles, *209*
Puborectalis sling around anorectal junction, *212*
Pulmonary abscesses, 171
Pulmonary artery(ies), 98, *176*, 188, *189*
  bifurcation of, 29
  bronchial artery and, anastomoses of, *70*
  coronary artery from, 127, *129*
  embolism of, 72
  exposure of, 44
  in cardiac transplantation, 138, *139*
  in pneumonectomy, 183, 184
  in tracheal resection, 193
  left, 81, 187, *188, 189*
  mobilization of, 160
  retrograde flushing of, 180
  right, *185, 186*
    vena caval attachment to, 100
  sheath of, 177
  subclavian artery and, anastomosis of, 44, 45, *46*
  tracheal compression by, 56, 57
  variations of, 177, *178*
Pulmonary embolectomy, 180
Pulmonary embolism, 72, 180
Pulmonary fissures, 167–168, *168*
Pulmonary ligament, 173
  accessory bronchial vessels in, 69
  in Blalock operation, 45
  in esophageal surgery, 222
  in tracheal resection, 193
  lymph vessels in, 182
    removal of, 219
Pulmonary lobes, 167–168, *168, 169*
  resection of, 173, 184–191
    bronchial arteries in, 180
Pulmonary lymphatics, 176, 180–183, *187*
  anterior and posterior views of, *181*
  overall view of, *180*
Pulmonary osteoarthropathy, 38
Pulmonary plexus(es), 153, 176
  in cardiac transplantation, 157
  vagal branches to, 187, *188, 189*
  in esophageal surgery, 223
  thoracic cardiac branches of, 156
Pulmonary segments, *168*, 169–170
  resection of, 173, 184–191
Pulmonary sequestration, 177, *178*
  extralobar, 209
Pulmonary valve, 118
Pulmonary veins, 98, *176*, 177
  anomalous, 112
  in mitral-valve replacement, 102
  in tracheal resection, 193
  inferior, *187, 189*
  intrapericardial course of, *179*
  right, 100, *101*
  superior, *185*, 187, *188*
  variations in, 179
  visceral drainage by, 72
Pulmonary venous hypertension, 108
Pulmonic stenosis, 69, 124, *125*
Pulmonic valve, anulus of, 103
  circumference of, 105, *106*
Purkinje's network, 132, 136

RADIATE LIGAMENT, *13*
Radicular arteries, 74

Radicular veins, 74, *75*
Rathke diagram, 53, *54*
Rectus abdominis muscle, in esophageal surgery, 222
  in pericardiocentesis, 164
Retro-aortic left brachiocephalic vein, 111–114, *113*
Retro-esophageal subclavian artery, 64, 81–83, *82, 84*
  arterial anomalies with, 42, 82, *83*
  as last branch of aortic arch, *41*
  obstructing, 56
  origin of, 54, *55*
  thoracic duct anomalies and, 231
Retrograde perfusion through coronary sinus, 147
Revascularization, cardiac, 141–152
Rhomboid muscles, *12*
  in cervicothoracic sympathectomy, 18
  in thoracoplasty, 10
Rib(s), cervical, approaches to, 8
  removal of, 7
  first, 3
    exposure of, 12
    neurovascular relationships at, *4, 11*
    posterolateral approach to, 10
    removal of, 6–8, *7*
  in coarctation surgery, 58
  regeneration of, 13
  removal of, for subclavian artery exposure, 45, *47*
    in thoracoplasty, 12
    through axilla, 6, *7*
  second, in cervicothoracic sympathectomy, 16
    removal of, 12
  third, in cervicothoracic sympathectomy, 19
  twelfth, removal in thoracic duct surgery, 233
Ring of Vieussens, 97
  damage to, 45
Roux loop in esophageal surgery, 219, 221

SAPHENOUS VEIN GRAFT, 149
Scalene approach, to mediastinoscopy, 35
  to mediastinotomy, 33
  to sympathectomy, 8
    cervicodorsal, 157
    to cervicothoracic, 16, *17–19*
Scalene fat biopsy, 35
Scalene fat pad, 33
Scalene lymphatics, 33, 182, 229
  metastasis to, 183
Scalenus anterior muscle, 3, *4*, 48
  in cervico-axillary extension of sternotomy, 50
  in cervicothoracic sympathectomy, 16, 17, *18*
  in mediastinotomy, 34
  in rib removal, 7
Scalenus medius muscle, 3
Scalenus minimus muscle, 3
Scalenus muscles, 3
Scapula, in thoracoplasty, 10, *11*
  vertebral border of, 10, *12*
Scapular nerve, dorsal, *12*
Scapular vessels, injury to, 49
Segmental artery, 170
Segmental bronchus, 177
Segmental vein, 167
Sequestration, pulmonary, 177, *178*
  extralobar, 209
Septomarginal trabecula, 118
Septum primum defect, 119
  atrioventricular node artery in, 146
  atrioventricular node in, *133*, 134
  closure of, 135

Septum secundum defect, 122, *125,* 126
  embryology of, 119, *120*
Serratus anterior muscle, 10, *11,* 12
Serratus posterior muscle, 12
Shumway technique of cardiac transplantation, *139,* 157
Sibson's fascia, 4, *5,* 6
  in apicolysis, 13
  in cervico-axillary extension of sternotomy, 50
  in cervicothoracic sympathectomy, 17, *19*
  in mediastinotomy, 34
Sinospiral muscles, *119*
Sinu-atrial node, 132, *133,* 134
  in atrial surgery, 100
  innervation of, 156
Sinu-atrial nodal artery, *144, 145*
  anomalous, 144, *145,* 147
Sinus venosus, 117, 119, *120, 121,* 122
Situs inversus, 66
  thoracic duct anomalies and, 231
Skeleton, cardiac, 103–106, *103*
  relations of viscera to, 199, *200–203*
Sliding hernia, 212, *213*
Søndergaard's canal, *101,* 102
Space of Burns in median sternotomy, 93
Sphincters, *211, 212*
Spinal artery(ies), 63, 73, 74
Spinal cord, blood supply of, 73–76, *75*
    interference with, 58
  border zone of, 74
  cervical, blood supply of, 63, 64
  injury to, 74, 75, 76
  intercostal artery division and, 59
  junctional zone of, 74
  sympathetic outflow from, 16
  thoracic, blood supply of, 65
Splanchnicectomy, approaches for, 206
  sympathectomy and, *20–23,* 24
  thoracic duct injury during, 232
Spleen, 205
  for coronary–extracoronary artery communication, 149
Splenic flexure of colon, 205
Stellate ganglion, 3, *4, 5, 155*
  in cervicothoracic sympathectomy, 16, *17*
    exposure of, 18, *19*
  removal of, 7
    for cardiac pain, 156
Sternoclavicular elevation, *49*
Sternoclaviculopectoral pedicle, 49, *50*
Sternocleidomastoid muscle, in cervico-axillary extension of
    sternotomy, 50
  in cervicothoracic sympathectomy, 16, *18*
  in mediastinotomy, 34
  in thoracic duct exposure, 231
  section of, 48
Sternocostal muscle, 151
Sternohyoid muscle, *155*
  section of, 48
Sternothyroid muscle, *155*
  section of, 48
Sternotomy, cervico-axillary extensions of, 49–51, *51*
  for thyroidal surgery, 78, *79*
  for tracheal exposure, 192, 195
  median, 93–99, *94*
    exposures in, 93–95
    for cardiac exposure, 100, *101, 109*
    for cervicothoracic exposure, 47, *49*
    for constrictive pericarditis, 164
Sternum, division of, 44
  retraction of, 93, 95

Stomach, 205. See also *Gastric.*
  anastomosis with esophagus, 206, 222–224, *224*
  cardia of, esophageal carcinoma and, 218
  in esophageal surgery, 219, 220, *221*
  in hiatus hernia, 212, *213*
  resection of, 72, 219
Stretch receptors, cardiac, 156
Subclavian artery(ies), 3, *4,* 63
  aberrant, approach to, 57
  bronchial branches of, 66
  cervical tracheo-esophageal branch of, 71
  esophageal branches of, 71
  exposure of, 45, *47*
  in rib removal, 6, 7, 8
  in thoracoplasty, 13
  left, exposure of, 44
    in coarctation surgery, 58, *61*
  origin of, *82*
  pulmonary artery and, Blalock anastomosis of, 44, 45,
    46
  retro-esophageal. See *Retro-esophageal subclavian artery.*
  right, bronchial branch of, 67, *69*
    origin of, 156
    thymic branches of, 86
  variations in, 40
  vertebral branches of, 41, 42
Subclavian lymph trunk, 182, 229
Subclavian vein, 3, *4,* 111
  in cervico-axillary extension of sternotomy, 50
  in mediastinotomy, 34
  in rib removal, 7
  in thoracoplasty, 13
  injury to, 48
    in mediastinoscopy, 35
  lymphatics of, 229
Subclavius muscle, in cervico-axillary extension of
    sternotomy, 49
  in rib removal, 6, 7
Subhepatic abscess, 199
Subhepatic space, 199
  approaches to, *205*
Subphrenic peritoneal relationships, *204*
Subphrenic space, 199
  approaches to, *205*
Subphrenic visceral relationships, 199–205, *200–204*
Subvalvular obstruction, 110
Sulcus terminalis, 117
Superior aperture of thorax, 3–9
  major relationships at, 3–6
Superior sulcus tumor, 34
Supernumerary bronchi, 177
Supraclavicular approach, to mediastinoscopy, 35
  to mediastinotomy, 33
  to sympathectomy, 8
    cervicodorsal, 157
    cervicothoracic, 16, *17–19*
Suprapleural membrane, 4, *5,* 6
  in apicolysis, 13
  in cervico-axillary extension of sternotomy, 50
  in cervicothoracic sympathectomy, 17, *19*
  in mediastinotomy, 34
Suprarenal gland, 199
Suprascapular vessels, 17
  injury to, 49
Suprasternal approach, to mediastinoscopy, *36, 37*
  to thymus exposure, 87
Suprasternal space, 36
  diverticulum of, 48
  in median sternotomy, 93

Sympathectomy, 16–24
  approaches for, 206
    extrapleural, 6, 10, *20*, 33
    supraclavicular, 8
  cervicodorsal, 156
    approach for, 157
  cervicothoracic, 16, *17–19*
    posterior extrapleural approach for, 18
  Linton's, *22*, 206
  lumbodorsal, 74
  thoracolumbar, *20–23*
Sympathetic ganglia, cervical, 153, *154*
Sympathetic nerves, cardiac, 153, *154, 155,* 156
  extrapleural approaches to, 33
Sympathetic plexus, blood supply of, 64, 69
Sympathetic trunk, *13*
  cardiac branches from, 153, *154,* 156
  collateral pathways for, 16
  dissection of, *22*
  extrapleural exposure of, *47*
  in cervico-axillary extension of sternotomy, 50
  in cervicothoracic sympathectomy, 16
  lumbar segments of, removal of, 24

TACHYCARDIA, 136
Tetralogy of Fallot, 124, *125*
  coronary anomalies and, 127
  interventricular septal defect in, *133,* 135
  surgery for, 129
    Blalock's, 44, *46*
Thebesian valve, 115
Thoracic aorta, descending, 63, 64
  development of, 53
Thoracic aperture, superior, 3–9
Thoracic artery(ies), internal, 15, 64, 86, 97
    communications with coronary arteries, 146
    course of, *94, 95*
    in Blalock operation, 45
    in coarctation surgery, 58, *60*
    in myocardial revascularization, 149, *150*
    in thoracoplasty, 13, *14*
    intercostal branches of, 65
    thyroidea ima artery from, 81
Thoracic duct, 29, 224
  anomalies of, 56
  collaterals for, 231
  exposures of, 231–233, *232*
  in cervico-axillary extension of sternotomy, 50
  in coarctation surgery, 59
  in esophagectomy, *223,* 224, 226
  in mediastinoscopy, 35
  in mediastinotomy, 34
  in vascular ring surgery, 57
  metastases to, 33
  normal pattern of, 228–229
  termination of, *230*
  tributaries of, 182
  variations of, 229–231, *229*
  vertebral artery and, 43
Thoracic esophagus, blood supply to, 69
Thoracic exposures, 44–47
Thoracic ganglion removal, 156
Thoracic lymph nodes, *14*
  removal of, *15*
Thoracic nerve(s), 3, *5,* 16
  root injury to, 12
Thoracic vertebrae, 12
Thoracic vein, internal, 13, *14*

Thoracic viscera, blood supply of, 63–77
Thoracic wall, 10–25
Thoracoabdominal incisions, 205–206
Thoracoabdominal structures, 197–234
Thoracolumbar sympathectomy, 20, *20–23*
Thoracoplasty, 10–13, *11, 14*
Thoracotomy, 44
  for Blalock operation, 45, *46*
  for cervicodorsal sympathectomy, 157
  for cervicothoracic sympathectomy, 16
  for esophageal surgery, 222
  for great vessel exposure, 45
  for heart surgery, 100, 108, *109*
  for intrathoracic goiter, 80
  for intrathoracic parathyroid tumors, 84
  for thoracic duct surgery, 232, 233
  for tracheal surgery, 192
  for vascular rings, 56
Thorax, superior aperture of, 3–9
  major relationships at, 3–6
Thymectomy, 87
Thymic arteries, 85
Thymic rests, 85, *86*
Thymic vein, 86, 95
Thymus, 29, 85–87, 95–98
  approach to, 93
  blood supply of, 64, *87,* 95
  exposure of, *47*
  in mediastinoscopy, 38
  in newborn, *85*
  in vascular ring surgery, 57
Thyrocervical arterial trunk, in Blalock operation, 45
  in cervico-axillary extension of sternotomy, 50
  in mediastinotomy, 34
  vertebral artery in common with, 42
Thyroid, blood supply of, 64
  cancer of, 78, *79*
  exposure of, 47
  goiterous, 78–80
  in mediastinoscopy, 38
  thymic rests of, 85, *86*
Thyroid artery(ies), 64, 71. See also *Thyroidea ima artery.*
  inferior, 63, 86
    anomalous origin of, 42
    in tracheal resection, 195
    recurrent inferior laryngeal nerve with, 83
    thymic branches of, 85
    tracheo-esophageal branches of, 192, *193*
      in esophageal surgery, 224
Thyroid veins, inferior, 72, 86
  in mediastinoscopy, 38
Thyroidea ima artery, *80–81*
  in mediastinoscopy, 38
  tracheo-esophageal branch of, 71
  variations in, 40, *81*
Thyroidectomy, 78, *79*
Trabeculae carneae, 118
Trachea, *187,* 192–196
  blood supply of, 64, 81
  cancer of, 195
  carina of, 170
    nodes of, 36
  cervical, blood supply of, 192
  compression of, 56, 57
  exposure of, 192–193
  goiter in, 80
  in mediastinoscopy, 36, *37,* 38
  injuries to, repair of, 192
  resection of, 193–195, *194*

Trachea (*Continued*)
  segmental bronchus from, 177
  thoracic, approach to, 93
    blood supply of, 69
  tumors of, 195
Tracheal arteries, 65, 70–72
Tracheal bifurcation, 29, *187*
  exposure of, 192, 195
  in bronchoscopy, 170
Tracheal cartilage, 195
Tracheobronchial lymph nodes, 36, *181*
  exposure of, 33
Tracheo-esophageal arteries, 71, 192, *193*
  in esophageal surgery, 224
Tracheo-esophageal fistula, *225,* 226
Tracheostomy, 192
  carotid arteries in, 41
  throidea ima artery in, 81
Transplantation of heart, 138–140, *139*
  collateral circulation following, 146
  innervation in, 138, 139, 157
  lymphatics in, 138, 139, 160
Transpleural drainage, *205*
Transversalis fascia, 93
Transverse foramen, vertebral artery entering, 42
Transverse process of vertebrae, in cervicothoracic
    sympathectomy, 19
  removal of, 12
Transverse sinus of pericardium, 98
Transversus muscle(s), in pericardiocentesis, 164
  in Vineberg procedure, 151
Trapezius muscle, *12*
  in cervicothoracic sympathectomy, 18
  in thoracoplasty, 10
Triangular ligament, left, 199
  in hiatus hernia repair, 216
Tricuspid valve, circumference of, 105, *106*
  fila coronaria of, *103,* 104
  septal cusp of, 115, *116*
  surgery of, 103
    atrioventricular block following, 117
Trigone(s), fibrous, of heart, *103,* 115
Truncus anterior artery, 184, *185*
Tumors, metastasis to scalene lymph nodes, 183
  parathyroid, 83–84, *84*
  paravertebral, 38
  superior sulcus, 34
  tracheal, 195

Ulcer, peptic, 216
Upper extremity, Blalock operation and, 45
  denervation of, 16
  pedicle exposure of, 10

Vagal plexus, blood supply of, 64, 69
Vagotomy, 216
Vagus nerve, 29, *187–189*
  in cardiac innervation, 153, *155,* 156
  in coarctation surgery, 58, *61*
  in esophageal surgery, 222, 223, *225*
  in patent ductus arteriosus, 57, *58*
  in pulmonary osteoarthropathy, 38
  in subclavian artery surgery, 57
Valvulae venosae, 119, *120*
Vasa vasorum, 98, 146
Vascular rings, 56–57, *56*
  derivation of, 53–56, *55*

Veins. See names of specific veins.
Vena cava, 97, 100
  catheterization of, 117
  in cardiac surgery, *101,* 102, 112
  in cardiac transplantation, 138, *139*
  in pneumonectomy, *183,* 184
  inferior, *116*
    pericardial attachments of, 102
    valve of, *116,* 117
      embryology of, 119, *120*
      fenestrated, *121,* 122
    orifice of, 117
  superior, 98, 134, *187*
    anomalous, 111–114, *112*
    in tracheal exposure, 192
Vena radicularis magna, 74
Venous ligation, venous return and, 48
Venous occlusion, spinal cord injury due to, 76
Ventricle(s), incisions into, 118
  left, in open heart surgery, 110
    in pericardiectomy, 164
    interior of, *105,* 108–110, *109*
  right, 115–123
    crista supraventricularis of, 118, 124
    double-outlet, 110
    hypertrophy of, 124
    incision into, 97
      transverse, 124, *125*
    interior of, 115–118, *116*
    outflow tract obstruction of, 118
Ventricular aneurysm, congenital, 210
Ventricular decompression, catheterization for, 110
Ventricular musculature, *103,* 118, *119*
Ventricular pre-excitation syndrome, 136
Ventricular septal defect, 124, *125*
  conduction elements and, *133*
  coronary artery variations and, 129
  repair of, 135
Ventricular septum, *105*
  as junctional zone, 141
Vertebra(e), transverse foramen of, vertebral artery entering,
    42
  transverse process of, in cervicothoracic sympathectomy,
    19
  removal of, 12
Vertebral artery(ies), *4,* 63, 74
  exposure of, 44, 45, 47
  in cervicothoracic sympathectomy, 17
  variations in, 40–43, *41, 43*
    retro-esophageal subclavian artery and, 82,
    83
Vertebral vein, *4,* 48, 72
  in cervicothoracic sympathectomy, 17
  in thoracic duct surgery, 232
Vertebrocostal foramen, 209
  hernia of, 178
Vieussens' ring, 97
  damage to, 45
Vineberg procedure, 149, *150,* 151
Viscera, exposures of, 199–207
  subphrenic relationships of, 199–205, *200–204*
  vasculature of, 63–77, *66*
Visceral veins, 72–73

Wolff-Parkinson-White syndrome, 136
Wrisberg's ganglion, 153, *155*